MENOPAUSE? HIT PLAY, NOT PAUSE!

A WISE WOMAN'S GUIDE TO "THE CHANGE"

GRACE ROSE

CONTENTS

INTRODUCTION

Menopause. Like death and taxes, the dreaded experience is inevitable yet woefully unwelcome. Many women are worried about the hot flashes, mood swings, vaginal dryness, and all the other undelightful symptoms of "The Change".

Whether you're noticing some of these changes insidiously creeping up on you or you woke up one morning to find yourself in someone else's body, my best advice to you is to learn about it and laugh about it. In fact, if you're feeling uncomfortable about discussing menopause, here's your chance to indulge every curiosity you may have about it. In the past, you see, the "Big M" wasn't talked about, so many women enter menopause completely unprepared for what could either be a wild ride or a lazy float down a sparkling river (okay, the lazy float probably isn't going to happen for most of us, but a girl can dream).

More than just exploring how to manage symptoms, I also want to give you inspiration. Our society may think we're "done" when we're menopausal, but we're actually just getting started on Chapter Wonderful. It's a benchmark in life when many women finally become who we were born to be. It's our time! And I'm not just saying that to deflect any dread, dishevelment, or distress. It's true!

A little educational, a little irreverent, and a little inspirational, this book is meant to help you see menopause in a positive light. Especially when it comes to your body.

Your body has served you so well and so lovingly for your whole life. She deserves to be loved, even if she's not as tight and perky as she was at 20. Come laugh with me as you enter this new stage of your existence!

Welcome to a very exclusive club. And let's face it: as we all know, menopausal women are hotter!

MY STORY

I was inspired to write this book to empathize, educate, and encourage all of us ladies experiencing something totally new happening to our bodies and minds.

My mother and grandmother were both 42 when they went through the meno, so after feeling strange things happen to my own body, I did a lot of research, and I learned that it tends to follow a genetic path. Great! (Sarcasm absolutely intended.)

After 17 years of being a physical education teacher in a secondary school, and physiology being one of the aspects that interested me the most, I was keen to do my own research into what and why things were happening to my body.

As I was only 40 at the time, I think I was in denial about actually beginning the menopause journey, so I decided to look into more holistic ways to ease my symptoms—which, by the way, had hit me like an express train to hell and seemed to appear overnight. Wonderfully delightful symptoms, such as:

Brain fog — not being able to actually speak words, or forgetting what I was saying part way through speaking with someone and having absolutely no sense of recall to be able to continue the conversation, even if they prompted me.

Night sweats — waking up in pools of water with wet hair (and even sweating from my arms and legs) and needing to change the bedsheets every morning

Blurred vision — black, floating clusters in my eyes that wouldn't go away

Itchy skin — my skin became so dry and itchy, and sometimes people would look at me oddly as I would act like a bear, rubbing my back up and down the nearest door frame

Urinary tract infections — or at least what I thought were UTIs. I had undergone months of investigations and scans on my bladder to determine the cause of the discomfort, as antibiotics weren't clearing up my symptoms

Anger —I hated being so constantly narky and angry all the time, and I seemed to spend the majority of my time apologizing to people I loved and cared about

I could go on and on here with all the symptoms, but instead I'll put a list of common ones associated with peri-menopause and menopause at the end of the book, along with a list of holistic remedies that are said to ease them.

For about 18 months, I used various online or over-the-counter holistic remedies, which, to be fair, *did* ease the symptoms, but only slightly. I'll share what I did, but first, I would like to acknowledge my doctor's gracious and essential help. I'm so grateful to my doctor for her approach, as I know of many people my age and younger who've been told by their GP that they're too young to be going through the perimenopause or menopause, which only leads them to suffer unnecessarily.

My advice is keep pushing, get second opinions, track your symptoms daily, and log your nutrition and daily exercise habits so that you can go to your GP armed with evidence to make them take you seriously. Unfortunately, menopause is still not commonly taught at medical school, and so many GPs have little knowledge about it.

I've created a symptom tracker/journal to help you show your doctors that the symptoms you're experiencing are linked to the menopause.

As I mentioned earlier, the aim of this book is to empathize, educate, and encourage all you ladies out there who are going through this new stage of your lives, and help you embrace it.

MENOPAUSE AND YOU

There's no doubt that menopause can have a significant impact on your quality of life for around, in some cases, a decade or so (now doesn't *that* sound like a party). A large study over nearly

9,000 women found that those who were experiencing menopausal symptoms reported lower health-related quality of life and higher work impairment. The most distressing symptoms included mood swings and joint stiffness. Surprisingly, hot flashes weren't the most problematic when it came to quality of life. The study's authors stated, "These findings suggest there is a humanistic and economic burden for women who reported experiencing menopausal symptoms. The results underscore the need for improved management of menopausal symptoms."[1]

Even a few years ago, menopause wasn't talked about in "polite society." Maybe it still isn't; I have no idea what duchesses and heiresses talk about at teatime, but I believe it's overdue that menopause gets the attention it deserves, and *not* as a syndrome or dysfunction.

Women need to talk openly about menopause, to drop our inhibitions, and be honest about what we're experiencing. Of course, talking to other menopausal women is extremely helpful, but we need to be able to discuss it with our families and partners, and even at work. We need to understand what the woman frantically fanning herself in the checkout line is experiencing, even if our initial instinct is to get the heck away from her, and quickly.

We also need to harness the collective wisdom of millions of women around the world who are sick and tired of being told that just because they've hit menopause, they're no longer desirable or contributing members of society. It's sad, but even some female authors on menopause still try to push the "Look like you're young and fertile!" approach. But menopause is not a disease or something you can treat. Yes, of course, you can treat uncomfortable symptoms, but the entire experience should be celebrated. Honestly.

Society is telling us that women should forever look 20, yet when we middle-aged women try, we're told to act our age. What are we supposed to do? Well, laugh, of course! When people give us funny looks if we suddenly sprint out of the room to splash cold water on our faces, what are we supposed to do then? Again, laugh! Humor makes big things seem smaller. Sometimes, of course, menopause is no laughing matter if you have severe symptoms and your quality of life has really gone down the toilet. I agree. Sometimes, all I want to do is curl up in a ball and make it all go away. With wine.

However, there are ways to make the experience more tolerable. Hey, life is messy. Menopause just turns the experience of living up a few notches. What I've discovered in my own journey is that there are women everywhere who are willing to lift you up and help you get through the hard parts.

It all starts with education. Education is the first step to improving your quality of life as you enter and go through menopause. Knowing what to expect and knowing your options for managing symptoms can take away a lot of the anxiety associated with any major change. But, more than just a clinical look at symptoms and treatments, let's look at the whole experience of menopause—woman to woman.

Journey with me through The Change. In this book, you'll read stories of real women with real menopause experiences (I've changed the names to protect their individual and very personal situations, but the stories are real. Their adventures and anecdotes will be in italics so that you can differentiate between their tales and the rest of this book). You'll learn what menopause is, why you're having symptoms, and how you can go through this chapter of your life in *style*.

Anthropologist and author Margaret Mead said, "There is no

greater power in the world than the zest of a postmenopausal woman." Amen! It truly is one of the most exciting times. When the media is focused on how horrible menopause is, let's focus on what it *isn't*: the end. It's not the end—*it's the beginning.* So let's approach it with a "bring it on" attitude!

WHAT'S THE DEAL WITH THESE "PAUSES"?

I t's bad enough having hot flashes at home.

"One morning (prior to me starting on the hormone replacement patches), my husband woke up in the morning convinced that I'd wet myself," says Elisa. *"Naturally, he was totally oblivious to the fact I'd been up all night tossing and turning and walking outside naked trying to cool down, not wanting to wake him in the middle of night to change the soaked sheets. You can imagine his relief when I explained that it was just from the night sweats and that I hadn't actually peed the bed!"*

That said, hot flashes at work can be even *more* embarrassing.

--Renee works in medical sales. A few years ago, her office was being renovated, so she temporarily used a desk near the IT guy who managed the company's database. She'd only experienced a few hot flashes before, but this one was like a volcanic eruption. Sitting there sweating with

what felt like a rush of hot lava in her veins, she said out loud, "Oh, crap! Power surge!", after which the IT guy jumped up and ran over, convinced that Renee's computer was completely fried (nope—just her insides). Embarrassed as she was about visibly melting in front of a 20-something guy, she couldn't stop laughing. Understandably!

This chapter tackles the stages of menopause, when they begin, how long each stage lasts, and provides a brief overview of the symptoms. It's good to know what's coming—and believe me, as my grandad used to say, "This too shall pass." Not that you can prevent hot flashes, which always seem to come at the least appropriate times, but at least they won't last forever.

And hey—I like to think of hot flashes as Mother Nature's way of lighting a fire under us to remind us that we're here to live life to the fullest!

WHAT IS MENOPAUSE?

There are four stages in a woman's reproductive life, and menopause is the end of your reproductive cycle. But, as you're about to see, it can also signal the beginning of an amazing new chapter of your life! Let's briefly delve into these cycles below.

Pre-Menopause

You're in your reproductive/childbearing years, having regular periods.

Perimenopause

This refers to the transitional time leading up to your last period and one year after your last period. Perimenopause may last 3-5 years on average, depending on your stress levels and overall health.

Your hormone levels are going just as mad as they did when you transitioned from girl to woman, except this time, the levels of estrogen and progesterone are dropping as your body shuts down the release of any remaining eggs. This is when you might start to experience symptoms that peak during menopause:

- Hot flashes and night sweats
- Shorter, more irregular periods
- Mood swings
- Sleep problems
- Lower sex drive (or higher, as you're about to find out)
- Vaginal dryness
- Brain fog
- Muscle and joint aches

You can still become pregnant during perimenopause (so beware!), though it's unlikely.

The symptoms of perimenopause are a lot less exciting for most women than when we first started menstruating. Back then, it meant we'd become women. Hello boobies, and hello boys! Everything was revolving around sex back then.

Now, with our childbearing years behind us, many of us feel "less" than we did in our prime. Becoming a woman opens up an exciting new world. We're taught that to be young and sexy is the absolute ideal we should all aspire to. The same with becoming a mother: we're valued by society when we procreate.

But nobody talks about the next phase. Many women feel an emptiness, because mature women tend to fade into the background and become invisible thanks to our culture, which does not revere or even respect women who are beyond their childbearing years.

However, your usefulness is *not* over. Please don't step to the sidelines and hide. Please believe me when I say that it's not "the end." It's just a new chapter, and that's what we're going to celebrate in *this* chapter.

Menopause

What's the definition of menopause? You're officially in menopause if you've gone a full year without a period. This *typically* happens anywhere between 41 and 61, with the average age being around 51. At this point, your ovaries have completely stopped production.

As you're about to discover, the classic menopause symptoms are *not* a given. Your stress levels and overall health have a lot to do with the existence and severity of menopausal symptoms.

Mila has some backyard chickens. She'd first got them just as the COVID lockdown started, thinking, "If I'm going to be stuck at home, I might as well get some chickens!" (Anyone else relate?) Of the original six, two lost their lives to predators, so Mila then added a handsome rooster and two younger hens. One of the original girls, Bee, was a champion egg layer. From the day this hen laid her first egg, she did not skip a day for two and a half years. Her eggs were always the biggest, and she even laid a double-yolker once. When Bee reached two and a half, Mila noticed that she was laying eggs with thinner shells, or sometimes no shells at all—just a weird sack that looked like a half-filled water balloon. Then Bee stopped laying eggs altogether, and her formerly large and bright red comb and wattles started to shrink. "She's going through *henopause!*" Mila realized. She officially retired Bee to a happy life of chasing the younger hens and digging up the garden.

Now, it's possible that this hen may have just taken a holiday (imagine—never taking a *single day off* for two and a half years?), and since it's winter as I write this, it's also possible that Bee may lay a few more come spring, since hens naturally stop laying when the days are short. But Mila thinks that Bee is going through menopause and that she's handed in her resignation as an egg-laying hen.

Not that I'm comparing anyone to a hen. I just found it amusing that hens' bright red combs and wattles shrink to pre-teen sizes and paleness when they stop laying. So we're not alone. Even animals go through The Change! Do you have any unspayed female pets who's gone through it?

Post-Menopause

Several years after all of this starts, your hormones are finally calming down, and you should be experiencing fewer (if any) symptoms as you transition from perimenopause to menopause. You may still experience occasional symptoms but, by now, menopause is a distant memory (thank you, *thank you*). The biggest concern during this time is that low estrogen levels are associated with a higher risk of heart disease, cancer, and osteoporosis. Great! (yes that's a joke once again).

Knowing what's going on in your body can help you come to terms with your symptoms.

WHAT CAUSES THE "PAUSES"?

Menopause can have natural causes or medical causes. Natural causes of menopause are hormonal. Medical causes can include surgery such as a hysterectomy, or medications such as chemotherapy that artificially induce menopause.

Causes of the Pauses: Natural Decline in Reproductive Hormone Production

Hormones are the body's chemical messengers. They coordinate functions like growth and development, metabolism, blood pressure, the sleep-wake rhythm, sexuality and reproduction, and even moods. Hormones are produced by the endocrine system, which consists of the pancreas, adrenals, thyroid, thymus, pineal, pituitary, testes, and ovaries. Some hormones, like estrogen, are also produced in adipose tissue (body fat).

Think of your hormones as musicians in a symphony orchestra. In the state called homeostasis, your hormones play in sync with each other and produce the beautiful harmony of a perfectly functioning body.

But have you ever been to the symphony and heard the orchestra warming up? It's discordant chaos! It's the same in your body. Or have you ever heard just one musician make a mistake? Even a small change in your hormone levels can have a big impact on the harmonious functioning of your body.

For the purposes of this book, we'll look at the three sex hormones present in the female body: estrogen, progesterone, and—to a much lesser degree—testosterone.

Each phase of menopause depends on changes in the body's natural production of estrogen and progesterone. This change corresponds with a decline in fertility. Did you know that women are born with a finite amount of eggs? Our bodies contain about six million during development as a fetus, about one million at the time of birth, and around 300,000 at puberty, but most of these never mature. During the reproductive years, we expel 400-500 (unfertilized) eggs during our periods. As we age, the decreasing number and quality of the remaining eggs influence fertility. As the body literally runs out of eggs, we enter menopause. (As I write this, I'm reminded of Mila's chicken and her "henopause." No more eggs! Bwaaak!)

Let's take a quick peek at the hormones that can go wackadoodle during *your entire reproductive life*. Womanhood is a wild ride, that's for sure.

Estrogen

Estrogen is one of the two reproductive hormones that make you female. It is considered the primary "female" hormone. Estrogen is made by men, too, just as the female body produces testosterone in small amounts.

There are three major types of estrogen:

- Estradiol: the primary form of estrogen present during your reproductive years
- Estriol: the primary form of estrogen present during pregnancy

- Estrone: the primary form of estrogen present after menopause

Estrogen plays several key roles in reproductive health. This chemical messenger signals your body when to begin and when to halt bodily processes that affect your sexual and reproductive health from puberty through menopause. It affects the development of secondary sex characteristics (boobs and curves, for example), fertility, and the timing of your periods. Estrogen is also responsible for maintaining vaginal blood flow, as well as vaginal elasticity and lubrication.

Estrogen has several important non-reproductive roles. It helps regulate blood sugar, cholesterol, bone growth, muscle mass, collagen production, brain function (including the ability to focus), and circulation/blood flow.

Most of your estrogen is produced in the ovaries during your reproductive years. It's also produced in much smaller quantities in the adrenal glands, and adipose (fat) tissue. also, your placenta secretes estrogen during pregnancy.

I mentioned earlier that even a small imbalance in the hormones can have significant effects. The disorders associated with estrogen imbalances include breast cancer, anorexia nervosa, amenorrhea (missed periods) or abnormally heavy periods, endometriosis, infertility, sexual dysfunction, obesity, polycystic ovary syndrome (PCOS), osteoporosis, vaginal atrophy, uterine fibroids and polyps, primary ovarian insufficiency, the dreaded premenstrual syndrome (PMS), and an increased risk of reproductive cancers. High estrogen, however, isn't a concern during perimenopause.

During perimenopause, estrogen levels decline—but not in a nice, smooth fashion. Oh no. Estrogen fluctuations are about as "hormonal" as it gets: they're on one day, off the next, can't make up their minds. It's pandemonium!

Most of the telltale signs of menopause correspond closely with declining estrogen levels: breast tenderness, hot flashes, headaches, brain fog, weaker and more brittle bones, irregular or no periods, chronic fatigue, trouble sleeping, mood swings, irritability, anxiety, and sexual discomfort due to vaginal dryness and loss of vaginal elasticity.

Progesterone

Progesterone is a sex hormone that's not produced by the ovaries. It's secreted by the corpus luteum, a *temporary* endocrine gland that is produced after ovulation—*every time you ovulate*.[9] (Crazy yet amazing, right?)

The job of progesterone is to prepare the uterus for pregnancy. It thickens the uterine lining, and it prohibits uterine muscle contractions that could cause the body to accidentally kick an egg out. If the just-released egg isn't fertilized, the corpus luteum dissolves and lowers progesterone levels, and you get your period. Since this book isn't about pregnancy, we won't go into how this amazing hormone makes your body a fertile garden for your growing baby, but it's worth looking it up online if you haven't already. It's fascinating!

Like estrogen, progesterone levels can become unbalanced. Low progesterone levels can lead to estrogen dominance, which can lead to abnormal menstrual cycles, infertility, and, if you do get pregnant, miscarriage or preterm birth.

Testosterone

Testosterone is also produced in the ovaries. It plays a role in the production of estrogen, and it may help maintain muscle mass and bone density. It's also linked to higher physical energy, mental focus, and libido.

So here's the interesting thing about testosterone: its production naturally declines with age, and this decline begins many years before perimenopause. In men and women, testosterone levels peak in our 20s and then start declining gradually. Testosterone production in the adrenal glands continues after menopause for non-reproductive purposes, but also declines with age.

This decline in testosterone raises an interesting question. Since testosterone has been declining in your body well before perimenopause started (when estrogen production declines abruptly), and the ovaries continue to make testosterone even after estrogen production has stopped completely, some researchers are saying that your *libido should not decline because of menopause, since libido is associated with testosterone.* One day, science will understand why our sex drive *really* fizzles during menopause; for now, however, it's linked to low estrogen.

Causes of the Pauses: Removal of the Ovaries

A medical cause of menopause is the surgical removal of the ovaries (oophorectomy). This causes abrupt, immediate menopause, because estrogen and progesterone are produced by the ovaries. Removing the ovaries is quite a shock to your system, and you may experience much more intense menopausal symptoms. Hormone replacement therapy is often prescribed to ease the transition.

A very small percentage of women experience ovarian insufficiency, in which the ovaries don't produce estrogen and progesterone in normal amounts. This can be genetic, or it can be due to an autoimmune disorder. Hormone replacement therapy is often prescribed until the natural menopausal age.

What about the removal of the uterus (hysterectomy) but not the ovaries before you naturally go through menopause? This procedure may be done if a woman has uterine fibroids that are causing abnormally heavy and persistent bleeding. This isn't menopause, however, because your ovaries are still releasing eggs and producing estrogen and progesterone. Wait your turn! Not to worry, though—it's a comin'.

Causes of the Pauses: Chemotherapy or Radiation

Cancer therapies may induce menopause. Chemotherapy can change menstruation and fertility, though this effect is sometimes temporary. Radiation that's directly aimed at the ovaries can affect their function, though radiation applied to other parts of the body (including the breasts) won't induce menopause.

IS IT MENOPAUSE?

If you're at the right age for menopause and suddenly having menopause-like symptoms, be aware that there are symptoms that could be menopause. Or they could be something else.

Depression, dizziness, cold feet, cold hands, headaches, hot flashes and night sweats, insomnia, irritability, and weight gain are normally thought of as classic menopausal symptoms.

However, they may also have nothing to do at all with "The Change".

Hot flashes, for example, could be caused by chronic stress or hormonal imbalances and not necessarily due to menopause. Insomnia, weight gain (particularly around the belly), brain fog, and mood swings can have dozens of causes also unrelated to menopause. If you're in doubt, get it checked out. Simple blood tests can determine this for you.

MENOPAUSE MYTHS

If you're breaking out in a hot flash just thinking about menopause, it's time to dispel some of the most damaging myths. Myths spread faster than gossip, and there are a lot of myths we need to send running off in shame!

Myth #1: Menopause is the Same for All Women

According to the 2015 study "Prevalence of menopausal symptoms among mid-life women: findings from electronic medical records" (Sussman et. al), the most common menopausal symptoms are NOT universal. Out of 102 patients assessed in the study:

- 40% experienced hot flashes (though Johns Hopkins University says it's closer to 75%)
- 17% experienced night sweats
- 16% experienced insomnia
- 13% experienced vaginal dryness
- 12% experienced mood disorders
- 12% experienced weight gain

The point is—don't assume that you *will* experience any or all the symptoms, or that they'll be severe! Many women don't have any hot flashes at all—they're still rockin' it in the bedroom, they haven't gained an ounce, and they're mentally sharp and emotionally calm. So don't be scared, just prepared.

There are many ways to cope with any symptoms you might have, but let me encourage you with these words: *don't expect the worst!*

Myth #2: Hot Flashes, Depression, Mood Swings, and Brain Fog Are Inevitable

The thing about this phase of our lives is that we often have lots of other challenging transitions happening at the same time: the empty nest syndrome with kids moving out, elderly parents who need help, maybe you're feeling stuck in a career that doesn't fulfill you, or perhaps you're going through an existential midlife crisis. The point is that anxiety, depression, and irritability are more common in this age range, but it's because of a massive pile-up of *life*, not necessarily hormonal changes.

Sleep problems often arise during menopause. But, again, the stresses of life could be causing them, so don't automatically assign the blame to menopause, tempting though it may be.

Brain fog is linked to hormonal changes, but it's also linked to natural aging, so saying menopause causes brain fog isn't an exact science. Consider this: how "busy" is your life and how overwhelmed are you? How many porcelain plates are you balancing at the same time you're juggling balls while trying to keep your dog from leaping after the balls? If you're like most of us, you've taken on a lot, so you can definitely be excused if some overwhelm creeps in. Your brain can only hold one thought at a time. When you're juggling so many things, and thoughts are competing for your attention, a few are bound to slip through the cracks. (I personally love the Notes and Voice Memo features on my phone. I use these to add a little order to my life!)

In the nutrition chapter, I briefly mention intermittent fasting, which is an incredible way to not only lose weight, but even reduce or eliminate brain fog and menopause symptoms. We'll get there in a bit, but for now, on with the myth busting!

Myth #3: It's Not Bad Enough to See a Doctor!

Most women experience mild to moderate symptoms. If your symptoms are bothersome, don't be a martyr. Don't diminish your quality of life by putting up with chronic brain fog, hot flashes that interfere with work or sleep, or chronic insomnia. There are ways to deal with all of these! It's better to keep your doctor in the loop with what's going on with you. Your doctor may prescribe hormone replacement, or suggest lifestyle modifications that will help ease symptoms.

Myth #4: You Need to Take Hormone Replacements

No! Hormone replacement therapy (HRT) is just one way to deal with bothersome menopause symptoms, particularly hot flashes. Acupuncture, exercise, meditation and other relaxation techniques, vaginal lube, and lifestyle changes can go a long way in easing symptoms. You don't necessarily need to resort to HRT.

But on the flip side...

Myth #5: Hormone Therapy Is Dangerous

Although it had an incredibly popular start, not that many years ago HRT was seen as a last resort, because it was linked to increased risk of breast cancer, cardiovascular disease, stroke, or blood clots. Today, doctors agree that HRT is an effective treatment for severe hot flashes. This can dramatically improve your life, and the key is to find a protocol that treats your symptoms without putting you at risk for serious disease. Your doctor will recommend the lowest effective dose and the most effective combination of estrogen and progesterone for your symptoms, and you'll be on HRT for the shortest time possible.

Do hormones ever return to normal after menopause? Yes—but it's a "new normal." Hormones will stabilize, which means your moods will become more balanced again. You may continue to have hot flashes for years, but less and less frequently. Women who choose not to have HRT can typically expect menopausal symptoms to last five to ten years or so.

Myth #6: You Can Kiss Your Sexy, Younger Body Goodbye

Things happen in your body as a result of menopause, but they're not all inevitable, and they're almost completely manageable. There's a lot you can do to keep your body functionally and aesthetically younger than your calendar years or your reproductive phase. We'll go into the symptoms and coping strategies later in the book.

Just remember this as you enter menopause: your body has been faithful to you all your life, and now it's time to show her some real love!

Myth #7: Menopause Is the End of Your Sex Life

Oh my goodness, no! While studies say that frequency of sex declines during menopause, sexual satisfaction often goes up. Could it be that we're just better at sex now? I think so! There could be plenty of other factors at play as well if you're experiencing lower libido: stress is one of them, or maybe your partner doesn't turn you on anymore. If you're experiencing vaginal dryness that leads to painful sex, it's natural that you'd want less of it! Talk about your concerns with your gynecologist and your partner. We all need to feel heard! We'll go into ways to spice up your sex life in Chapter 7, because the end of reproduction shouldn't mean the end of fun!

Also, some women's sex drive actually *increases* during menopause. We'll deep dive into this in Chapter 7!

Myth #8: You Can't Get Pregnant

Oh yes, ma'am, you can! While fertility declines as you enter perimenopause and you have highly irregular periods, you can still get pregnant. Although you're much less likely to get pregnant after 45 as your periods start being irregular, pregnancy can still happen. Doctors recommend continuing with birth control until you're officially menopausal, when you haven't had a period for 12 months straight (the official definition of menopause, as mentioned previously). If you're just now entering perimenopause, keep tracking your cycle so you know when you're officially menopausal.

Myth #9: You Will Gain Weight

Nope! Well, not necessarily. While declining estrogen levels may change the placement of any fat you gain (around your middle, rather than the hips and thighs), the real culprits of midlife weight gain are a slower metabolism due to loss of muscle mass, as well as a more sedentary lifestyle. If you make exercise and healthy eating a priority, you can stay at your ideal weight through menopause and beyond.

Myth #10: You Will Go Through Menopause When Your Mother Did

Yes, genetics matter, but so do other factors. Smokers will go through menopause sooner than nonsmokers. Autoimmune disorders, as well as any surgeries or medications that change estrogen/progesterone production, will also put you into menopause earlier.

Myth #11: Menopause Starts in Midlife, After You're 40

For most women, yes. The average age of the start of peri-menopause is 51, but perimenopause can also happen in your 30s or even 60s!

Myth #12: Menopause Lasts "Forever"

When you're in it and you're having strong symptoms, it can sure feel that way! The average duration of menopausal symptoms is seven years. For some, it can go on for twice that long. Or you might be done in two years. It partly depends on genetics and partly on lifestyle. Smoking and drinking make symptoms more severe, and they'll last longer. Stress is another huge contributor to the severity and duration of symptoms. Exercise and relaxation techniques make the symptoms better, and may also shorten the duration of menopause.

Myth #13: You're Old Once You've Been Through Menopause

Define "old"! In the Middle Ages when the average life expectancy was 40, today's menopausal woman would already be long gone. In fact, she probably would've died in childbirth. While menopause is a major transition, you don't have to think of your age in numbers. If your perimenopausal symptoms started in your late 40s, it doesn't mean you're "done" before you hit 60! After all, isn't 50 the new 30? Many women experience a resurgence in vitality after menopause—a time when they can finally be themselves!

Myth #14: You'll Develop Urinary Incontinence

Bladder tissue thins during menopause, which makes urinary incontinence a problem for some women but, again, not *all* women. Kegel exercises and vaginal estrogen creams can most certainly help.

Myth #15: If You Had Surgical Menopause, You Won't Have Symptoms

False. A total hysterectomy, or surgical menopause, involves the removal of the uterus, cervix, ovaries, and fallopian tubes.

The drop in hormones is drastic upon removal of the ovaries, and hormone replacement therapy is almost always prescribed to ease the symptoms. You can definitely expect to have symptoms just like you would if menopause had come naturally!

Incidentally, some people believe it's a myth that men have menopause, too, but it's actually a real thing. It's called andropause, and it corresponds with significant decreases in testosterone. However, the guys have it easier—their hormones don't fluctuate with as much drama as ours! They don't experience the hormonal roller coaster; testosterone just kind of fizzles away with no drumroll and no fanfare. At least we women have a little bit of excitement with our journey, for better or for worse.

Now that we've dispelled the myths, let's talk about what actually happens in your body during perimenopause and menopause.

2

WHO ARE YOU AND WHAT HAVE YOU DONE WITH MY BODY?

Evelyn likes to laugh about what she calls the Seven Witches of Menopause: Ouchy, Bitchy, Sweaty, Sleepy, Chunky, Foggy, and Moody. "Today, Sweaty came and stayed for a while. Then suddenly she was gone and in came Foggy and Moody. I think Chunky has moved in permanently. So has Ouchy, and my husband isn't a fan of her. Sleepy has been making an appearance once in a while, but at least I'm not seeing much of Bitchy!"

Aside from the famous hot flashes, a lot goes on in a woman's body during menopause. Many of these changes aren't exactly pleasant, but they are manageable.

Many women develop a negative body image during menopause, because society values youth and it sexualizes women. These normal body changes have benefitted an insanely profitable cosmetics industry, as women desperately turn to Botox, surgery, and rivers of serums in an attempt to defy time.

But honestly—the happiest women I know have embraced the changes going on in their bodies.

Sure, they reminisce about when they were younger, thinner, and had firmer skin. But they also stop dyeing their hair and flaunt the silver fox look. They adjust their fitness routines to better care for their bodies. They become more attuned to their bodies and nourish themselves with good food and exercise, and, most of all, *they refuse to stop living.*

YOUR CHANGING BODY

Menopause can be a strange thing. Your body seems different, even if you don't have all the classic menopause symptoms. Knowing what happens in your body when you become "a woman of a certain age" can help you be prepared.

Notice that I used the words "in your body" and not "*to* your body." It's important that you don't feel like a victim of menopause. It's a natural change. It can absolutely not be fun at times, but it's not happening *to* you. It's happening *in* you, and it's perfectly normal. A positive attitude can go a long way in easing the emotional impact of menopausal symptoms!

Changes in Your Period

As your ovaries start slowing and shutting down the release of eggs, you'll notice fluctuations in your period. This is usually the first symptom women notice. Periods may become irregular, heavier or lighter than usual, they may last longer than one week, may go away for months before coming back, and you may have spotting.

When Jacquie hit 42, her periods went crazy. They'd last off-and-on for weeks. Sometimes she'd bleed for three weeks straight, and then nothing for two months. It turned out that uterine fibroids were causing the excess bleeding—not menopause. Because of the fibroids, Jacquie had a partial hysterectomy (which did not usher in menopause); her perimenopausal symptoms began at 49. No matter your age, it's important to talk to your doctor about any changes in your period. They may be related to menopause, but maybe not!

You can expect that your periods will likely be all over the place, with no rhyme or reason. This can make things a bit complicated if you're trying to avoid getting pregnant, which, as already mentioned, you still can even though your fertility has dropped and many eggs are no longer viable. I recommend talking to your doctor about continuing with birth control during your perimenopausal years.

Hot Flashes and Night Sweats (or "I'm Still Hot, It Just Comes in Flashes!")

Recently, Barbara was at a Christmas gathering that included several people her age, as well as their children—all millennials. Suddenly, Barbara turned beet red and blurted out as she fanned her face with her hands, "I'm having a hot flash!" One of the millennial women turned just as red, as if she was the one having a hot flash, and she looked absolutely mortified. Every one of the "older" women had a little laugh about it. I see this story as an example of how wonderful it is to be a mature woman and no longer care what other people think!

Hot flashes and night sweats are the biggest complaints many menopausal women have. The hypothalamus, the brain's temperature regulatory center, is influenced by estrogen. When declining estrogen levels make the hypothalamus malfunction, blood vessels near the surface of the skin dilate, increasing blood flow. As a result, you may feel like hot lava is coursing through your veins—the feeling can be all-consuming, but sometimes manageable. You may feel chilled, dizzy, or nauseous. Your face may turn red, you'll probably sweat profusely, and your heart rate will spike.

Ironically, a hot flash is actually meant to cool you down! Lower estrogen levels make your hypothalamus hyper-sensitive to the slightest change in body temperature, particularly at night when estrogen does a lot of the temperature regulating. The temperature gauge in your hypothalamus suddenly thinks you're too warm, so it initiates a hot flash to get you to sweat. Unfortunately, in this case, the cure is worse than the problem! I have yet to hear of a single woman saying she felt "too warm" in the moments before a hot flash.

Emily was at a restaurant enjoying dinner with her college-aged daughter. Suddenly, she turned crimson red, and rivers of sweat started pouring down her face. There was no hiding this eruption. Emily pressed a glass of ice water against her neck until the hot flash burned itself out, while her daughter fought desperately to keep from laughing hysterically. "Just you wait…" she hissed.

Some women experience alternating sensations of heat and cold. Some experience a crawling feeling on the skin, or even nausea just prior to a hot flash.

Katie says she always feels hot flashes coming on. At first, it feels some-thing like a strong hunger pang with some nausea. She calls it a "hor-mone dump". Within 30 seconds, she's on fire. Emily says she never feels them coming—they just hit her like a flame thrower.

Some women experience "cold flashes" where they feel chilled. Whatever your experience, it's not a one-size-fits-all phenomenon.

Most hot flashes last from 30 seconds to five minutes. For some women, hot flashes don't feel like "flashes" at all. Some-times, these unwelcome bursts may feel as if you left for work when it was freezing outside. You turned up the thermostat to "Sahara Desert in the summer at noon" and left, and when you came home, you walked into an oven!

How frequent your hot flashes are, how long each episode lasts, and how many years you'll have them is, of course, highly individual. The average is seven to ten years, but the most intense hot flashes and night sweats seem to happen earlier in perimenopause.

Your stress level has a lot to do with the severity of your flashes, and some women find that caffeine and spicy foods make them even worse. Imagine—one less cup of coffee or forgoing that tamale might just lighten your load. Maybe not, but experimenting couldn't hurt!

Changes in Muscles and Bones

Many women notice a loss of athletic performance during menopause.

First, there's loss of muscle mass. Estrogen plays a role here as well, thanks to its influence on apoptosis. Apoptosis is the natural death of cells as part of the building/renewal phases that all tissues undergo throughout your lifetime. Estrogen signals cell building, so when its levels decline, cells don't renew as quickly or as often. This is why low estrogen can lead to a loss of muscle mass and bone density. Bone density naturally decreases by 0.5-1.5% during perimenopause and menopause. Some women may experience drastically higher losses in bone density, as high as 3-5% annually.

It's unfortunate but normal to have less skeletal muscle strength as we age. We know that as testosterone levels gradually decrease in men, it contributes to loss of muscle mass and an increase in fat mass. The key here is gradual. But what about in women? Estrogen contributes to muscle strength, and as it declines rather dramatically during menopause, so does muscle strength, especially after age 55.[2]

Joint Stiffness and Pain

There are estrogen receptors all throughout the body, including the joints. As estrogen levels drop, there's less of an anti-inflammatory effect on the joints, which can add to pain and stiffness. Try supplementing with turmeric (curcumin, the active ingredient in turmeric, acts like a natural anti-inflammatory and may reduce pain).

Another normal part of aging is a gradual breakdown of the cartilage and synovial fluid in the joints, which can lead to pain and eventually osteoarthritis. Even very athletic women may find it harder to perform repetitive motion activities such as bicycling, or to get up effortlessly and painlessly from sitting on the floor.

The combination of less muscle mass and stiff joints leads many women to exercise less. Even though it may be harder and hurt a little more, *don't ever give up on exercise* or you'll enter a vicious cycle that will lead to frailty and loss of mobility. Reducing exercise leads to even more muscle loss, loss of flexibility, weight gain, and accelerated loss of bone density.

Less exercise is the exact opposite of what your body needs to remain vital through your menopausal years. Instead, you could find a personal trainer who can help you with exercises that don't hurt but continue to challenge your bones, muscles, and connective tissues to stay strong.

Weight Gain

Nancy says, "I keep looking at myself in the mirror thinking, 'I'm out of shape.' Well, round is a shape!"

Many women's bodies start shapeshifting during menopause. Where there was once no belly, now there's a paunch. Where there were once firm thighs, now there's jiggle. Where there was once a shapely waist, there's now a shapeless blob. Where there were once perky breasts…

This shift is partly due to a loss of muscle mass, which slows the metabolism and encourages weight gain, and it happens to coincide with menopause. It's also due, in part, to decreases in testosterone and estrogen levels.

What's really maddening is that menopausal fat gain tends to accumulate on the belly. Continuing with an exercise program and improving your dietary choices can help you stay trim and fit your entire life. We'll go into nutrition and exercise for menopausal women in later chapters.

Changes in the Skin

Part of aging involves reduced collagen and elastin production, again due to declining estrogen levels. Collagen is a protein that makes up about 80% of your skin and is responsible for its firmness. Elastin is the protein that helps your skin bounce back after being stretched. A loss of collagen and elastin leads to softer, saggier, and less elastic skin. Your skin may also feel drier than normal. I recommend using high-quality body and facial oils or moisturizers to trap moisture in the skin. Collagen powder supplements and a diet rich in micronutrients can also help.

In addition, you may notice an increase in actinic keratoses, or dry, scaly patches of skin. These are the aftermath of the loss of pigment-producing melanocytes and yes, they're often precancerous, so keep your skin covered when you're out midday. Be sure to get these checked out and removed ASAP before they turn into cancer!

Changes in Your Scent

You may also notice a change in your natural fragrance. An individual's unique scent is closely related to the state of their gut, so any changes to the gut microbiome, whether induced by diet or hormonal fluctuations, can change your scent. The amount of pheromones you secrete also changes in menopause, which can also alter your scent—more on that in the sex chapter!

Changes in the Heart

You may feel heart palpitations start to happen during menopause. You may also experience increased heart rate, especially during a hot flash. These are generally nothing to worry about, but be sure to get regular checkups and consult your doctor if you're worried about them.

Heart disease is another concern for some postmenopausal women. This is partly due to a more sedentary lifestyle (again, due to the no-fun aspect of working out with less muscle mass and more painful joints), but heart disease can largely be prevented with positive lifestyle changes even as estrogen levels drop.

Changes in the Breasts

Often, as estrogen levels fall, so do the breasts. You may notice less breast fullness and increased tenderness. Breast sagging is partly due to the weight of the breast tissue and partly to decreased muscle tone. Exercise and weight management will help keep the girls perky.

But what about the Big C? A woman's risk of breast cancer increases to about one in 28 after menopause, but lifestyle changes can help. This means limiting alcohol, eating nutritious food, maintaining a healthy weight, being physically active, and using HRT wisely.

Hearing Loss

Did you know that the inner ear has estrogen receptors? I didn't either! This means that estrogen also affects balance and hearing. If you notice hearing loss, definitely get it checked out. HRT could help if hearing loss is related to menopause.

Vertigo and Dizziness

Like many female-related issues, there's not much research on why menopausal women often complain of vertigo and dizziness. Here's what we know so far.

Benign paroxysmal positional vertigo (BPPV) is characterized by a sudden spinning or off-balance sensation, like motion sickness. Vertigo can develop due to changing hormone levels, and it's fairly common in perimenopausal women. Osteoporosis may also be a factor in developing BPPV.

Dizziness is a sudden sensation of lightheadedness, disorientation, or feeling "woozy." Both this and vertigo can be symptoms of menopause. Estrogen receptors in the inner ear mean that estrogen plays a role in balance. Therefore, lower estrogen levels may contribute to feeling like you're in someone else's body at times.

Anxiety can also contribute to vertigo and dizziness (dizziness is actually a physical symptom of anxiety). Heart palpitations and dehydration can lead to dizziness, as well. If you experience vertigo or dizziness frequently, be sure to get it checked out. Dizziness can be caused by low blood sugar, low blood pressure (standing up too fast), or other factors. Vertigo, on the other hand, can be caused by stroke or a tumor.

Manage stress and avoid caffeine, alcohol, tobacco, and sugar to minimize dizziness and vertigo.

Thinning Hair

Hair grows more slowly and often thins with age. Everyone's hair is different, but even women with formerly thick hair (and lots of it) may find that they're losing more than usual as they go through menopause. Red light therapy and topical hair growth creams can help stimulate the hair follicles to spend more time in the hair growth phase. At this point, you may consider a different haircut that takes emphasis away from the thin spots and onto your facial features.

One place that you'll likely see more hair is the upper lip and chin. This is due to very gradually declining levels of testosterone and abruptly declining levels of estrogen. As soon as there's more testosterone in your system than estrogen, you may develop secondary male sex characteristics, which seem to be largely confined to facial hair. Oh, joy! But unfortunately, it likely can't be helped. You may find yourself plucking or waxing your upper lip and chin as you go through menopause. Don't shoot the messenger!

Decreased Bone Density

Estrogen regulates bone cell metabolism, or the creation and breakdown of bone tissue. It promotes the activity of osteocytes, osteoblasts, and osteoclasts, which are the cells that make new bone tissue and reabsorb old bone tissue. Lower estrogen levels mean that the body isn't making as many bone-building cells; basically, we reabsorb more bone tissue than we make. Eventually, this leads to brittle and weak bones.

A diet rich in calcium, protein, vitamin D, and fat (because vitamin D is fat-soluble!) will help. Weight-bearing exercises, running, resistance training, yoga, and dance will put just enough stress on your bones to stimulate new bone formation.

Worsening Sex Life

Some women experience vaginal dryness during menopause, which can, as one would think, lead to painful sex. Some women also experience a lower sex drive.

Vaginal atrophy (sounds so sad, doesn't it?) can manifest as vaginal dryness and recurring urinary tract infections (UTIs). Lube, Kegel exercises, and more sex can help (having more sex will keep your vaginal muscles active). More on spicing up your love life in Chapter 7!

Poor Bladder Control and Urinary Tract Infections

As the pelvic floor relaxes, you may find yourself experiencing incontinence in the form of a little dribble when you laugh or sneeze. UTIs are also common, and you can try drinking cranberry juice if you want an effective natural remedy. Kegel exercises will help tone the pelvic muscles.

Gum Disease

Can menopause really cause bleeding gums? Unfortunately, yes. Estrogen is an anti-inflammatory. As it declines during menopause, your body loses some of that protection and doesn't do as good of a job taking care of oral irritants, such as bacteria, that cause periodontal disease.

What's ironic is that poor dental hygiene also leads to chronic inflammation, which interferes with hormonal balance throughout the body. It is now known that periodontal disease (red, swollen, bleeding, and receding gums) are an indicator of other inflammatory disorders that have nothing to do with the mouth: metabolic syndrome, autoimmune disorders, cardiovascular disease, and osteoporosis.

If you have any problems in your mouth, get them checked out and boost your oral hygiene. When you think about it, your mouth is a gateway to your body. Taking care of that gateway is critical to your overall health!

Poor Gut Health

Further down the digestive tract, low estrogen levels can also change your gut health.

Menopausal women are more likely to have irritable bowel syndrome (IBS), which includes gas, bloating, stomach pain, gas, diarrhea, or constipation.

Why is gut health so vital? Because it's the driving factor for your overall health and wellbeing.

Sex hormones affect the health of the trillions of bacteria that live in the digestive system. Most of the time, these bacteria (called the gut microbiome) find their own balance. But chronic inflammation, hormonal fluctuations, and poor diet can upset this balance. This has immediate and long-term consequences to your overall health. The ancient Greek physician Hippocrates wasn't wrong when he said that all disease begins in the gut!

Hormonal imbalances, and particularly the decrease in

estrogen and progesterone, can affect the speed at which food moves through the digestive system. Sometimes, this decrease can cause bowels to empty faster, which leads to diarrhea, nausea, or stomach pain. Sometimes, it can cause the opposite, where food moves slowly through the gut, causing gas, bloating, and constipation.

And it works both ways. A healthy gut influences the production of sex hormones!

Refer to the nutrition chapter for ways to keep your gut microbiome healthy. And, of course, if you notice anything unusual going on with your digestive system—especially if you notice blood in your stool—get it checked out immediately. [3]

Sleep Disturbances

Sleep problems become more common in menopause. Night sweats, stress, and other menopausal symptoms can make it hard to fall asleep and stay asleep. If you have difficulty falling asleep, or you wake up in the middle of the night and have trouble falling back asleep and routinely feel sleepy during the day, you may also be suffering from anxiety, depression, irritability, and poor focus as a result of not getting enough sleep.

Why does menopause disrupt your sleep? Well, estrogen helps regulate body temperature at night. It also regulates serotonin production, which affects your mood and gives estrogen a mild antidepressant effect. Once estrogen levels drop, you'll feel more stressed and may have trouble sleeping.

You may also develop sleep-disordered breathing, such as sleep apnea or snoring (fabulous, right?). I'll share some great tips for sleeplessness, because getting enough zzzz's is vital to your health.

As women age, our circadian rhythms tend to shift, too. We may get tired earlier in the evening (but resist going to bed at "children's hour"), and yet we also tend to wake up earlier. And with various sleep disturbances, we may become chronically sleep deprived.

YOUR CHANGING BRAIN

Hormonal changes affect memory, moods, cognitive function, and focus. It's important to realize that the mental and emotional symptoms of menopause are as real as the physical symptoms. Remember, a little hormonal fluctuation can have big consequences. If you're struggling and need help, don't wait. Getting help is a sign of strength!

One of the things that you'll "enjoy" about The Change is that it's okay these days to talk about it! It's no longer seen as a disease or a disorder, but rather as a normal part of life.

Yes, there are some annoying things that can happen to your brain, like "Kitchenheimer's" (where you go into the kitchen and immediately forget why). Speaking of which, I saw a funny post on social media not long ago. Unfortunately, I don't know the author, but it really hit home:

"*I realized I had to use the bathroom.*

I got up and walked across the house to the pantry.

I couldn't remember why I was in the pantry.

I remembered I had to use the bathroom.

I walked across the house to the bathroom.

Sitting on the throne I remembered why I went to the pantry.

Toilet paper."

I'll be the first to admit that there's nothing funny about becoming forgetful. It's scary. I do my best to laugh about it, but the truth is that sometimes I feel that my brain is misfiring like it did when my pre-teen hormones were raging and my neural synapses hadn't quite fused into what we know as a functioning adult brain. And now that I'm middle aged, I'm worried about dementia and Alzheimer's.

Our partners and friends may notice, so have a conversation about menopause with your loved ones, because not everyone knows that menopause can contribute to brain fog. Some partners may say that menopausal forgetfulness is a convenient excuse for everything. Now we all know that it isn't—but for a few years at least, you can play the menopause card and nobody will dare put you down for brain fog!

Mood Swings

"As I go through menopause, I've come to terms with something," says Miriam. *"I'm done trying to make everyone happy. I've been doing that my whole life. It's hard. I'm tired. But pissing them off—that's easy. Just wait five minutes, and Angry Miriam will come out!"*

Mood swings are another unwelcome symptom of menopause. One minute everything is puppies and rainbows, the next minute you want to lash out in anger, the next you're dissolving in a puddle of tears, and then the clouds lift and you're happy again. It's incredibly frustrating!

As I've mentioned, heightened emotions may have more to do with overwhelm and with the fact that menopause is a sign that much of our lives are behind us. And that's a tough pill to swallow.

One thing to be aware of is that true depression (persistent low moods) is not solely due to hormonal changes during menopause. Hormonal changes can cause mood swings, but not clinical depression. While menopause can increase your *risk* of depression, it isn't a direct cause—and depression is something that should be professionally treated so that you can have a good quality of life.

Brain Fog

To make light of a not-always-funny subject, below are some real-life examples of brain fog.

--"*Just last week, I was meeting my friend for lunch, and we found ourselves discussing brain fog,*" says Linda. "*I was trying to give her tips that had helped me. However, during the short time it took the waitress to place our meals on the table, neither of us could recall anything we'd just been talking about! Frustrating, but we had a good laugh about it.*"

--*Rachael tells a funny story. "I'd just finished a little snack of carrots and hummus, and on the way to the kitchen, I tried to put them away—in the China cabinet! I stopped myself at the last minute, feeling oddly puzzled as to why there were teacups in the fridge. 'Oh. It's not the fridge...'"*

"*A funny incident happened to me just this last weekend,*" laughs Katerina. "*I filled my dishwasher soap compartment with washing up liquid, only to come back to a kitchen flooded with bubbles!*"

You may find yourself struggling for the right word (and make up a nonsense word instead!) and forget names, tasks, plans, schedules, and commitments. I can't emphasize enough the need for lists. Either write them down on paper or use the Notes feature on your phone to save yourself the frustration. Of course, remembering to even *look* at the list is challenging enough sometimes!

Headaches and Migraines

If you're prone to headaches and/or migraines, they may worsen during menopause. Most women who don't often have headaches may not notice any change in this area. Be sure to stay well-hydrated, since dehydration is a common cause of headaches and your brain literally shrinks when cells don't have enough water. Spending more time in nature has been proven to help as well, as the color green actually has a soothing effect on our nervous systems. Fact!

THIS, TOO, SHALL PASS!

What a depressing list of symptoms, right? But let's not dwell on it! If you even have them at all, you may be blessed with the "mild" versions—and in any case, they're not forever!

The best thing you can do is to take excellent care of yourself, and I'll outline steps to do just that in later chapters. And who knows, it might not even be that bad for you!

Natalia says, "I was one of the lucky ones. I was happy when my periods stopped, because I didn't want any more children. I didn't mourn the loss of my periods—in fact, I was more energized without the monthly blood and iron loss! My symptoms were all manageable. What's best about my situation is how great I felt when it was all done. I sleep well, I have so much energy, I only have an occasional hot flash when I'm stressed, I feel more like myself than ever, actually—more confident and self-accepting."

Start this new chapter of your life with some new goals and a good attitude. Let's build on that frame of mind now!

3

ACCEPTING & LOVING YOUR NEW BODY

Sophie looked in the mirror one day, as she'd just experienced a hot flash upon getting out the shower. "I've become my mother!" she cried out in dismay.

Many women will ask, "How do I get my old body back?" The answer is—you can't. At least not completely, although there's a lot that you can do to slow the aging process. The more energy you put into not aging, the more stressed you'll be and the faster you'll age. Pretty counter-productive! Stress is a big factor in rapid aging, so one of the best ways you can learn to accept your changing body is to try not to stress about it.

I love the story of triathlete and American Senior Olympian Sister Madonna Buder, who is affectionately known as the "Iron Nun". Sister Madonna is now 92 and still breaking records, mostly for being the oldest competitor out there. She holds the world record as the oldest woman Ironman finisher (the

Ironman triathlon is considered to be one of the world's most difficult one-day sporting events). But she wasn't always a triathlete. When she was 48, Buder was told that exercise is a way of improving the mind, body, and spirit, and of bringing calmness and tranquility. She started training, completed her first triathlon at 52, her first Ironman at 55, and she shows no signs of stopping!

So don't give in to any excuses like, "I'm too old." No, you're not. Just because your body is closing up shop on making babies doesn't mean it's used up! And besides, many women find that once they've actually gone through menopause, they have more energy because they're not bleeding every month. That may be an icky way of putting it, but hey—it's definitely true, and it's definitely good news.

LEARNING TO LOVE YOUR NEW BODY

You can focus on changing what you can change, such as exercising more to prevent loss of muscle mass, eating healthy to support your body at the cellular level, managing stress, and getting enough sleep. Support your body in being healthy, strong, and vibrant, even if it looks different than when you were 20. And if you haven't been active in your younger years, it's not too late to start!

Speak Kindly To and About Your Body

I'm a firm believer that our bodies listen very carefully to what we say about them, and they respond in kind. It's not the words, necessarily—it's the emotions behind them that have a very real and direct effect on our cells. Whether this is too woo-

woo for you or not, it can't hurt to stop saying things like, "I hate my thighs" and instead focus on how grateful you are to have thighs that let you experience life!

Refrain from saying negative things about your body, even if your body is no longer tight and perky. Love your body with kind words. Admire your good qualities. Don't worry about the rest, because, honestly, who told you that older women aren't beautiful? Society, that's who! And now that you're old enough to make up your own mind about beauty, isn't it time to stop idolizing the young and firm, and start worshipping the inner beauty that comes with age, grace, and wisdom? I think so!

In fact, go and do this right now: go smile at yourself in the mirror for two minutes. It's going to seem weird at first, but very soon even the most forced smile will turn into a genuine one, and you'll literally feel joy coursing through your body. Most of the time, you'll even burst into laughter! Two minutes every day of smiling at yourself in the mirror—while mentally saying, "I love myself" (or "I love you", if you prefer)—is an amazing self-love practice that changes your brain chemistry and makes you feel *so good*!

Love What Your Body *Can* Do

Focusing on what your body can do and not on what it can't starts with seeing your body as a faithful instrument that does its very best to help you experience your life.

Back when you were 20, your body was a cute little sports car. She was fast, she was shiny, and she had curves in all the right places. Now, some 20-30 years later, she's not as shiny as she once was. Maybe she needs more frequent tune-ups. Maybe she needs her oil changed more often. Maybe she needs a few expensive repairs. Maybe she's in the shop longer than you'd like.

But is there anything sexier than a vintage car? It's rare! It's beautiful! It's an exhilarating, head-turning ride! Imagine taking a ride in a vintage automobile down a winding seaside road, sunglasses on, the wind in your hair, your favorite song playing loud… You don't care at all that she has some miles on her. The engine really starts humming once a car is broken in and has a few miles on her!

Strength Train

Strength training will help more than any other type of exercise in keeping your body looking great. It will give you defined, sexy muscles, a flatter tummy, toned arms, and a tight booty. Even simple body weight exercises like the plank, squats, and pushups will do wonders for your physique!

Give Yourself a Wardrobe Makeover

It's no fun staring at a closet full of clothes that don't fit. Get rid of them! They're yesterday's style anyway. Treat yourself to a chic new wardrobe. I'm not suggesting you go out and spend thousands on the latest trends. Instead, opt for a few timeless, elegant pieces that you feel good in, and round out your collection with a few items you'll want to wear every day—again, pieces you feel good in whether you're going to work, making a grocery run, or walking the dog.

Less is truly more. We all tend to wear the same six or seven outfits all the time anyway, especially if nobody is looking! So you might as well upgrade to six or seven chic outfits that make you feel elegant, and donate the rest.

Don't go for a "sexy" look only because sexiness is (unfairly!) associated with youth; go for elegance—a look that most younger women can't pull off without the poise that comes with age!

Get Off the Scale

How much you weigh can weigh heavily on you (pun intended). However, is that all there is to you, a couple of extra pounds? The numbers on the scale truly don't matter. All they do is stress you out!

Besides, muscle weighs more than fat, so prioritize building muscle mass, which will naturally shed fat in the process.

What matters more is how you feel, how much energy you have, how strong and flexible you are, how much endurance you have, and how your clothes fit. Focus on what you can change through a healthy diet and exercise.

Strength training, healthy eating, stress management, and even intermittent fasting can do wonders for a belly that wasn't there before.

And while a wardrobe change might be in order, settling for shapeless muumuus and kaftans isn't the answer. Don't hide your body, because that only contributes to feelings of shame and low self-worth. There are lots of wonderful resources in magazines and online that can help you dress for your body type without looking frumpy. Forget "dressing for your age" if you're comparing today's menopausal woman to your mother's or grandmother's generation. Sixty is the new forty!

Move Those Bones! Fight Gravity!

You can change the type of exercise you do, but whatever the case, *don't stop moving.* Yoga, tai chi, and Pilates are great ways to maintain or build muscle mass and flexibility as you age, without putting undue stress on stiffer joints.

If you want to fight something, don't fight age—fight gravity! Resistance training will keep your boobs and booty high and firm, and your bones and tendons strong. Find a fitness trainer to help you set and achieve fitness goals—and enlist another menopausal woman to join you as a fitness buddy! They say that misery loves company, but so does motivation!

Love Your Beautiful Face!

Smiling is so good for your body, your brain, and your attitude. Nothing makes an "older" face more beautiful than a smile. In fact, smiling more will give your face a radiant glow.

The best thing you can do for your skin is to *stop eating sugar* and drink more water. Sugar causes inflammation that ages skin faster. Indulge your sweet tooth with dark chocolate or fruit, but avoid junk sugars (more on this in the nutrition chapter).

When it comes to water, one gallon (or about four liters) of water daily will keep your skin feeling firmer and plumper while keeping your organs functioning smoothly.

Love the stories that your wrinkles tell. Every one of them has a tale. Some of them you might not want to hear ever again, but it's your stories that make you who you are, and they're what make you so interesting. People want to hear stories from interesting people, not from plastic people with no evidence of ever having made facial expressions! Smiling—I believe, anyway

—gives you good wrinkles. Laughter and good company are the best things you can do to improve your attitude during menopause!

If your skin is drier than it used to be, use a high-quality skin oil or a moisturizing cream to trap moisture and keep your skin supple.

Perk Up, Ladies!

It's time to become really good friends with the girls. Regular breast inspections and immediate action on any weird stuff like dimpled or puckered skin, lumps, or changes in skin tone can help you kick cancer's butt (should it ever appear).

Love the girls and perk 'em up with resistance training. Building up your pectoral muscles will support and lift your breasts!

You Silver Fox, You!

A couple of years ago, young women in their 20s started embracing the "granny" look by dyeing their hair ash gray. I found that very funny! Little did those chickies know…

Whether or not you're graying, you can improve hair health by avoiding excessive shampooing (twice a week is ideal) and using gentle, natural hair care products.

I recommend you show yourself some real love by saying goodbye to hair dye. I know it's a big, intimidating step, but I guarantee you'll say, "Why didn't I do this sooner?" Many women were forced to quit dyeing their hair during the pandemic lockdown when hairdressers were shut down, and now they *love* it. Finally, no more expense, no more hassle, better hair and scalp health…and it's one of the many ways to declare to the world, "Yeah, I'm not a spring chicken anymore. I'm a woman. Hear me roar!"

One of the reasons to ditch the dye is to make your hair look fuller. If your hair is dyed dark and it's thinning, the contrast between your scalp and your hair can make your hair seem even thinner. Gray hair doesn't contrast the scalp, and thinning hair will look fuller.

Get a stylist to create a big, softly blended area so that you don't have to deal with the dreaded gray tide moving slowly away from your scalp. And then just forget about it (though it might take a few months to a year to completely grow out the faux you). You might even notice how much healthier your hair looks when you stop dyeing it, you gorgeous silver fox!

Don't Sweat the Hot Flashes

Love yourself through the heat! You'll probably wash your sheets more often than ever, and who doesn't love climbing into a fresh, clean bed? You'll save a lot of money on heating bills—a *lot* of money. And you'll also detox your body through sweating!

Aside from drinking a glass of ice water or going outside to cool off, try deep, slow breathing to calm your nervous system. Inhale deeply through your nose and feel that cool air rushing into your lungs! Then exhale slowly and deeply through your mouth, taking no more than five to seven breaths per minute until the flash cools down.

Treat yourself to some super-soft, extra-large, highly absorbent beach towels to lie on in bed. And remember a nice soft towel for your pillow, too!

Anne got in the habit of having a spritz bottle filled with water in every room. When she had a hot flash, she'd spritz her face and torso with water, and let evaporative cooling work its magic.

Sweet Dreams!

Some women find relief for insomnia through hormone replacement therapy, which we'll talk about next. You may also get some relief with antidepressants.

If you don't want to go "full pharma" on your sleep disorders, here are some tips that can help you get a good night's sleep:

- Melatonin is the sleep hormone, and it can be found as an over-the-counter medication. These supplements may cause gastric distress in some women, so take the lowest effective dose.
- Cognitive behavior therapy (CBT) involves working with a therapist to recognize the thoughts that negatively impact your sleep, and replace them with more positive thoughts that don't cause sleep-wrecking distress.
- Avoid any caffeine or nicotine after lunch. And hey—stop smoking altogether.
- Reduce stress. Meditation, relaxing activities, a bath, reading, hobbies, soothing music, and gentle movement like stretching can help you prep your body for sleep.
- Get your magnesium! Many women are chronically deficient in magnesium. If you have restless legs or muscle cramps, try supplementing with magnesium.

It also helps with heart rhythm and other functions, and it's said to promote sleep, as well.

- Avoid alcohol. A glass of wine with dinner is fine, but more may contribute to insomnia.
- If you do wake up at night because of night sweats, keep the lights off, don't reach for your phone, and don't get up. Keep a glass of cold water on your nightstand to cool your body internally, and have a change of clothes handy so you don't lie there soaking wet.
- Keep your bedroom dark and cool. A fan will help keep the air moving.
- Listen to a sleep meditation track or soothing sleep music if you wake up at night. If you sleep with a partner, get some headphones for this purpose.
- Maintain a healthy weight. Obesity is associated with sleep disorders, including sleep apnea.
- Stay well hydrated during the day and drink a full glass of water *at least* one hour before bedtime. A hydrated heart is a happy heart that doesn't have to work as hard to push thick blood (dehydrated blood) through your body. You'll sleep better—as long as your last evening drink of water isn't too close to bedtime!
- When you're burning up in the middle of the night, breathe in slowly and deeply through your nose. Imagine the cool air moving through your nasal passages into your lungs. Exhale slowly and deeply through your mouth, and imagine letting all that hot air escape.

- Follow a regular sleep schedule. Go to bed and get up at the same time every day, and, wherever possible, avoid napping during the day. Cat naps of ten minutes are generally okay, but longer ones will keep you up at night.
- Take CBD oil. CBD is a chemical found in marijuana, but it doesn't contain THC, so you won't get high. Besides being used as a sleep aid, CBD is also said to help with aching joints and anxiety.

"CBD is the only thing that works for me," says Kat. "It doesn't knock me out like a sleeping pill. It's not addictive. I sleep better than a baby because I don't wake up every two hours screaming. That's what babies do. I have a laugh every time I hear people say they sleep like a baby— obviously whoever says that has never had babies screaming all night!"

Get Help

Even though menopausal symptoms are normal, if they're getting in the way of your life and work, get help.

Seeking help isn't a sign of weakness. It's a sign of strength and it's a sign of self-love.

Products that claim to "fix" the symptoms of menopause are everywhere. Some work and some don't, so you'll want to have a talk with your doctor. Let's start with a treatment that can give many women relief: hormone replacement therapy.

HORMONE REPLACEMENT THERAPY (HRT)

"One Friday morning I was training in the gym with a couple of my friends," says Jessica. "We were having a moan about how bloated and

frumpy we felt, along with laughing at the ridiculous things we'd said or done that past week. Our brains and bodies seemed somewhat out of our control. One friend said she'd been to see a 'menopause doctor' who'd been very empathetic, and explained that what was happening to her body was a result of a dramatic drop in estrogen levels.

"I booked in with the same doctor, who was so understanding and spoke to me with just the right amount of 'scientific jargon' and 'layman's' terms to help me grasp what was happening to me and my hormones. Voila—this was the first stage of accepting it wasn't my fault that these things were happening and that there was a reason why I'd been a complete bitch to everyone around me!

"Initially, I was against HRT due to all the old-school horror stories about putting loads of weight on and getting breast cancer. This doctor did explain all the risks and possible side effects, but they were outweighed by the positive effect HRT could have on my body.

"I've now been on HRT patches (estrogen) and take progesterone tablets before bed, which have the added bonus of helping me sleep. I was continuing to struggle with UTI symptoms, so the doctor prescribed me some topical estrogen cream that I use twice weekly. I can honestly say my bladder hasn't felt this relaxed for a long time.

"My mood is now so much more stable, my brain fog has lessened, and I no longer get night sweats. I'd be lying if I said I didn't still experience the symptoms to some extent, but I'm aware that we're dealing with hormones here and that finding the balance may take some time."

If you have severe menopausal symptoms, your doctor may recommend HRT with the aim of restoring premenopausal levels of estrogen and progesterone. Aside from relieving hot flashes, vaginal dryness, mood swings, low libido, and other menopausal symptoms, HRT can also help prevent osteoporosis.

The benefits of HRT are believed to outweigh the risks, but this therapy isn't for everyone. It's not recommended for women with a history of breast cancer or any other reproductive system cancer, a history of high blood pressure or blood clots, or women with liver disease.

You might have heard some crazy stories about HRT, so let's dive into its turbulent history.

In 1929, American biochemist Edward Adelbert Doisy discovered the hormone estrogen, and in the years that followed, researchers delved into what it and other hormones do.

In the 1960s, Dr. Robert Wilson wrote a book called *Feminine Forever*. In it, he claimed that menopause "is a hormone deficiency disease, curable and totally preventable; just take estrogen." Wilson convinced millions of women that menopause wasn't natural, and that estrogen replacement was the only way to, basically, remain a woman (read: attractive and desirable).

What's perhaps most annoying and troubling about Wilson's book is that menopause, a completely natural process, was now seen as a disease. Wilson wrote that with estrogen replacement, a woman's "breasts and genital organs will not shrivel. She will be much more pleasant to live with and will not become dull and unattractive." He was basically saying that menopause was a problem *for men*. Aw, the poor dears—such an inconvenience for them that their wives are going through menopause! What a way to make a woman feel awful about herself, when there's absolutely nothing wrong with her.

Now, personally, I'm a fan of HRT because it helped me cope with strong menopausal symptoms. What really bothers me, however, is the patronizing way Wilson portrayed a woman's worth by sexualizing her and implying that she's only desirable if she's young, beautiful, sexy, and doesn't show the slightest signs of age. That sexist approach was the prevailing attitude back then, unfortunately. Even today, there's such a high value placed on youthful beauty that society completely misses out on the inner beauty and wisdom that can only come with age and experience.

HRT popularity peaked in the 1990s, but then plummeted after HRT was found to cause more harm than good, including being linked to endometrial (uterine) cancer.

The Women's Health Initiative study that caused the uproar about the link between HRT and endometrial cancer fed an incredible media frenzy that scared many women away from HRT. The study was later re-analyzed, and new research states that HRT is safe for most women. However, the public remains unconvinced. That's unfortunate, because a lot of women are suffering needlessly simply because they (or their doctors) don't want to touch HRT with a barge pole.

Here's what we know. New studies have found that, for most women, HRT has more benefits than side effects. When doctors started lowering estrogen doses and combining estrogen with progesterone (to better mimic the body's natural hormonal balance), the risk of uterine cancer went down. This was confirmed by the Nurses' Health Study (Goldstein et al, 1996), which observed nearly 60,000 women as they went through menopause. The researchers concluded, "We observed a marked decrease in the risk of major coronary heart disease among women who took estrogen with progestin."

Today, HRT is once again increasing in popularity, and not just as a treatment for hot flashes. It can improve your sex life, and it's even used as a preventative treatment for the most common diseases affecting postmenopausal women.[4]

The North American Menopause Society, The American Society for Reproductive Medicine, and The Endocrine Society are all in agreement that healthy menopausal women can safely use HRT to get relief from symptoms.[5]

- Low doses of vaginal estrogen (as a cream, ring, or suppository) are an effective treatment for vaginal dryness
- Higher estrogen doses, along with progesterone, are used to treat hot flashes; women who've had a partial hysterectomy (uterus removal, but ovaries intact) can take estrogen alone
- Using a combination of estrogen and progesterone HRT for five years or less is generally recommended; beyond that, there's an increased risk of breast cancer (although estrogen alone doesn't appear to increase breast cancer risk)
- Both estrogen and estrogen/progesterone HRT increase the risk of blood clots in the lungs and legs, which is similar to the risk brought on by birth control pills, rings, and patches

What Are the Types of HRT?

There are two different types of HRT. Traditional HRT uses manufactured hormones from synthetic sources, while bioidentical hormone therapy (BHRT) uses hormones from animal or plant sources. According to the Mayo Clinic, bioidentical hormones aren't safer or more effective than traditional HRT.

The word "bioidentical" means that, chemically, the hormones are identical to the hormones naturally produced by the body. These same chemicals can be reproduced artificially, rather than from plant or animal sources.

Your doctor can advise you on which is better for you.

Systemic hormone therapy may come in topical and inserted versions and contains a high dose of estrogen. Systemic HRT is used to treat common menopausal symptoms like hot flashes.

Low-dose hormone therapy includes vaginal products that secrete low doses of estrogen. This is used to treat vaginal problems and urinary incontinence.

Within these two types, there are also differences in dosage and hormone ratio. Your doctor will help you choose the one that's right for you based on your symptoms.

- Most women use a combination of estrogen and progesterone
- If you've had a partial hysterectomy (uterus removed but ovaries intact), you may be given estrogen only
- You may take HRT orally or as a skin gel, implant, vaginal cream, skin patch, or intrauterine coil
- There are different treatment protocols, including regular use or HRT taken in cycles, depending on whether you're taking estrogen only, estrogen/progesterone, and your individual dosage

When Can You Start HRT?

You can start HRT as soon as you begin experiencing

menopausal symptoms (I'll get out of the way as you rush to the phone to call your doctor).

Typically, most women start with a low dose, and you may not feel the effects for several weeks (so don't go running back to the doctor and say it doesn't work unless you've given it up to three months to take effect). If you're still not experiencing relief after the first three-months, your doctor may increase your dose or change the type of HRT.

How to Stop HRT

HRT is used only until menopausal symptoms pass, which is typically a few years. However, the longer you take it, the higher your risk of breast cancer. Once you're ready to stop, you can choose to stop abruptly or gradually. Most women wean themselves off HRT gradually, which can help those dreaded hot flashes from making an encore appearance.

Side Effects of HRT

As with any medicine, HRT may cause side effects in some women, which can include vaginal bleeding, breast tenderness, nausea and indigestion, headaches, and abdominal pain. These symptoms usually stop several months after starting treatment.

You can reduce side effects and potential risks by working with your doctor to determine the best product and the most effective delivery method. For vaginal-only symptoms, many women prefer low-dose estrogen products. Doctors recommend always taking the lowest effective dose for the shortest possible time to minimize long-term risks.

ALTERNATIVES TO HRT

If you're having strong menopausal symptoms but can't or don't want to take HRT, there are other ways to get relief, and we'll examine them below.

Lifestyle Modifications

There are non-pharmaceutical routes to managing menopausal symptoms. One way to manage hot flashes is to lower the thermostat and sleep with your window open or keep a fan near your bed to keep things cooler at night.

Go Natural

One of my favorite ways to cope with hot flashes is to wear layers of clothing made from light, natural fabrics. It may surprise you that wool is actually a great choice! These days, many wool clothing options, including T-shirts and undergarments, are incredibly soft, lightweight, and breathable. They also dry a lot faster than cotton garments, so you won't feel cold and clammy after a hot flash. For women who like to sleep in the nude, I recommend sheets made from natural fabrics that wick moisture away from the body. Carry an extra T-shirt around with you (or whatever's work-appropriate) to change into in the event of an epic hot flash.

Stop Smoking

Stop smoking—for a million reasons, including the fact that smoking tobacco has been linked to early menopause.

Manage Stress

Stress can make your hot flashes worse and much more intense. Stress spikes your cortisol production, which further messes up your delicate hormone balance. Cortisol, which is one of the stress hormones, basically prepares your body for the fight-or-flight response, whether the danger is physical or emotional. It spikes block progesterone and estrogen receptors, so even if your body is producing enough progesterone and estrogen, you might experience symptoms of low levels of these hormones. And if your body is already producing less estrogen and progesterone, chronic cortisol spikes will amplify the symptoms.

If you're chronically stressed, I recommend yoga, meditation, self-care, prioritizing your to-do list, reducing caffeine, and getting plenty of fresh air and exercise.

Breathwork

Ever heard of box breathing? It can help you cool your body and relax your mind during a hot flash. Breathe in through your nose on the count of four, then hold for four, then exhale through your mouth for four, and finally hold for another four. Repeat. Imagine the cool air entering your body and the hot air leaving.

Antidepressants

Your doctor may prescribe certain antidepressants to treat your hot flashes. This can be tricky, because some antidepressants can lower your libido even more. However, some of the newer antidepressants don't have this effect at all.

Acupuncture

Traditional Chinese medicine (TCM) is based on promoting the natural flow of life force energy, or Qi (chi), in the body. Whenever there's a blockage in the body and Qi becomes blocked or stagnant, that means there's too much in some areas of the body and not enough in others. This can affect hormone balances.

Acupuncture can be a way to suppress hot flashes and night sweats, improve moods, help with heart palpitations, ease joint pain, irregular or heavy periods, and painful periods.

Testosterone

Strange as it seems, taking testosterone (which the ovaries also produce in small amounts) as a gel or cream can improve energy, mood, and sex drive. Since testosterone is partially responsible for estrogen production, it may raise your estrogen levels slightly. It likely won't do much to ease your hot flashes, but testosterone supplementation can make you feel better overall. And, no, it won't make you grow a moustache!

4

LOVING YOURSELF THROUGH
THE CHANGE

L ike anything, menopause is what you make it.

Evelyn was having a New Year's Eve celebration with her younger sister Marie. It was an incredibly cold night, at least twenty degrees below freezing, which is crazy cold regardless of whether you measure in Celsius or Fahrenheit! The ladies happily sat by the fire sipping mulled wine, laughing and telling stories. Suddenly, Evelyn turned bright red. She jumped up, flung open the door, and stepped out into the frigid night. And then she took off her top, stripping down to her bra! Marie couldn't believe her eyes. What was Evelyn doing? Evelyn just stood there in the freezing mountain air wearing nothing but her bra, her breath steaming. After a few minutes of calmly standing outside, basically half-naked in weather that would give a normal person frostbite, Evelyn calmly put her blouse back on and came indoors. As Marie sat there with her jaw on the floor, Evelyn laughed and said, "Hot flash." Later that evening, Evelyn walked Marie to her car, this time bundled up like an Arctic explorer. "Geez, it's freezing out here!" Evelyn shivered.

She stood shaking beside Marie's car as Marie struggled to start the engine in the bitter cold. After a few groans of protest, it finally roared to life and Marie was off. Marie texted Evelyn later to say she'd gotten home safely, and Evelyn replied that she'd just enjoyed another half-naked romp under the stars! Marie felt like she'd spent the evening with a Tibetan monk who was able to sit in the snow for hours in deep meditation, clothed in nothing but flimsy robes. 'What magical superpower was this?' she thought to herself. Three years later, Marie experienced her first hot flash. Finally, she deeply understood why Evelyn had needed to step outside to cool off!

Did Your Positive Attitude Leave with Your Period?

Attitudes can alter greatly during The Change. Many of us wish we didn't look like we do. We recognize that more of our life is behind us than ahead of us. It's natural to become depressed, anxious, or angry with our own mortality staring us in the face.

Some women avoid the inevitable, some fight it, and some accept it. I think we all go through each of these in no particular order. One day we dress decades younger because we remember how sexy we felt then. The next day we hit the gym with every ounce of energy we have, because that belly fat isn't responding to our diets. And the next day we relax with a good friend over a cup of tea and a slice of cake, and laugh at menopause stories.

There are some things you can do to slow the aging process, like exercise and nutrition. The key to aging gracefully, though, is to change what you can, accept what you can't, and make the most of the precious time you have.

Be Here Now and Don't Overthink It

If menopause changes are causing you stress, try to be in the moment. Don't think about what's ahead or behind—only what's going on now. Remember that you're entering a new phase in your life, when it's not all about your body and your looks, but rather about your heart and your soul. Your body will still be along for the ride, even if it doesn't look like it did 20 years ago.

The truth is that this very moment is the only one that matters, because it's the only moment that exists. Yesterday is a memory. Tomorrow is imaginary. *Only right now is real.* What can you do right now to make your life more interesting, exciting, happy, peaceful, loving, and an endless list of other qualities that bring a smile to your face and make you jump for actual joy? This moment is precious. In the face of strong emotions and physical symptoms, you can still learn to put your focus where you want it: on creating an amazing new chapter of your life!

Be Okay with Your Feelings and Feel All the Feels!

I'm making light of menopause, because I find that laughter truly is the best medicine. That isn't to say that feelings of anxiety, frustration, dread, sadness, or even anger don't ever come up. Of course they do!

However, here's the key: don't diminish the importance of menopause, but at the same time, don't make it bigger than it is.

I'm a firm believer that where your attention goes, your attention grows. The more you focus on how awful menopause can be, the worse it *will* be. The more you focus on the joys of menopause, the better it *will* be.

The thing about feelings is that they come no matter what, and if you don't dwell on what caused them, they will go. Allow yourself to fully experience your feelings. Feel all the feels! Here's a beautiful exercise I discovered that can help you when you're overcome with strong emotions.

When you feel a strong emotion, pull your attention away from the thought that created that emotion, such as the anxiety, frustration, anger, and sadness that can come from thinking, "I'm embarrassed about my body." Put all your attention onto the physical experience of the emotion, which is really nothing more than an electrochemical reaction in your body. How does it feel as these chemical signals go through your body in response to a thought? Do you feel a constriction in your chest, a pit in your stomach, muscle tension, a heaviness, sweaty palms, or tears? Just keep focusing on the experience of the emotion. Within 90 seconds, it will pass and you'll feel calm again. Once this happens (and it will if you don't keep going down the rabbit hole of thinking about how much you hate your body!), show your body some love.

You can repeat this exercise anytime. It's okay to feel what you feel! If you suppress your feelings, they can come back at the worst possible time. Until you process what's on your mind and in your heart, those feelings will keep coming back to visit you again.

Carrie is a biologist who was diagnosed with breast cancer at age 29. She went into chemically induced menopause as part of her treatment. She says, "I struggled so much to let myself grieve. I mean, every possibility of my becoming a mother to my own biological child was taken away from me. For years, I'd try to push away the anger and the grief, but then I noticed that when I just let myself cry and without thinking that I should be over it by now, I felt better."

Carrie's story is different from most women who go through natural menopause, but that doesn't mean those of us without a life-threatening disease don't feel the loss. We grieve, too, and grief doesn't follow a timeline. You can't just cry it all out one day and then be okay.

"For me," Carries continues, "moving forward means being okay with my feelings. If I try to push them away, they always come back—usually when it's extremely inconvenient! So I just sit with them until they ease up, and then I try to have a good laugh. I think that other women also experience tough feelings about menopause. It doesn't matter if it comes naturally or chemically. I try to transform the grief into laughter. Every time I tell my story, if I can help just one woman relate, then I've done my job."

She ends with, "Mourn, but don't wallow. It's okay to mourn the passing of your reproductive years! And, by all means, if you do feel the need to mourn, take all the time you need. Mourn on your schedule, in your own way."

I agree. Don't wallow. Just because the reproductive part of your life is over is no excuse to plop yourself on the couch with a tub of ice cream and binge-stream romantic chick-flicks for the rest of your life. After all, you lived a fulfilling life before you had your first period. You can love this new part without it!

Repeat after me: sixty is the new forty. Let it become a mantra of sorts, because it's 100% the truth.

Practice Gratitude

Say thank you to your body. Thank it for the experiences it's given you. Thank it for its faithful service. Isn't your body amazing? Go beyond looks for a minute. If you really take the time to think about just how much work your body does every day without any input or guidance from you, performing with such remarkable efficiency and precision to keep you alive and to let you experience life, do you think this knowledge would change the way you relate to it?

You may not have been given the body that you consider ideal. And it may have changed significantly, or be in the process of changing, due to menopause.

However, you can do a lot with your body to bring it closer to your ideal, through exquisite self-care. Especially now, when your body could really use some TLC for all the hard work it did throughout your reproductive years!

Surround Yourself with Supportive People

The beauty of being a mature woman is that we're far less prone to caring about what other people think. Honestly, if they're talking about your looks in a disparaging way, then you can really see just how shallow and petty they are, and how their own insecurities are coming across as ugly criticism. In other words, what they say is a reflection of them. It has *nothing* to do with you!

Surround yourself with people who see the real you—people who don't care that you have jowls or that you've put on a few pounds. People who genuinely care about you literally do not see your body as flawed. They can see past the physical aspects of you, because they are aging too, and they accept it. These are the kinds of people you can always talk to if you're feeling bad about yourself.

"Menopause has given me the green light to be myself," says Tina. "I have no time for drama anymore. No time for energy vampires, negative nellies, or anyone who says 'yes, but...' whenever I say something positive. I've invited all of them to sail away from my island of serenity."

Laugh About It

Classic brain fog! If you haven't experienced menopausal brain farts yet, they're on their way. And there's nothing to do but laugh about it. Some comical examples:

Debbie recalls, "The other day, my husband found the kitchen surface cleaner in the fridge, that I'd obviously put in there at some point..."

And Jamie told me about this gem: "A few weeks ago, I was shopping and was heading back to find my car in the car park however, it wasn't there. I phoned my husband to tell him the car had been stolen, and he told me that I had been dropped off by my friend that morning!"

It's true what they say about laughter being the best medicine, so let's have a laugh about the perks of menopause!

Michelle says, "I said to my sister the other day when she was complaining about her whiskers, 'What whiskers? I can't see any, but then again, my eyesight isn't what it used to be.' We had a pretty good laugh about it."

This next little bit of joy isn't so much funny as it is a cause for celebration: you never have to worry about birth control again! So who cares what other people think? You have now achieved wise goddess status. You can turn the thermostat down and save *so much money* on heating bills! You never have to worry about ruining white linen dresses with your period! You can wear whatever you want and do whatever you want, and if people call you eccentric, hooray! You can be moody and blame it on menopause! (Just kidding; don't be moody. Be passionate.)

Life has given you an incredible richness of experiences and wisdom, and the more you accept yourself now, the more you'll greet the world with a radiant inner glow that makes those hot flashes and wrinkles completely irrelevant.

Talk to Your Family

Let them know what's going on. Prepare your loved ones (let them read this book!) so that they understand what's different about you and why. That way, you'll go through menopause feeling understood. If they're embarrassed to talk about it, you can start with something like, "It's like a snake shedding its skin" or "It's like being on a roller coaster and I never know what's coming next." Help them understand that unless you're going through it, you can't really know what it's like and, honestly, that you don't know exactly what it will be like either! Ask for patience and empathy. Let them know that "this too shall pass", and tell them what they can do to help.

Normalize Menopause

It's not a disorder, syndrome, or disease. It's as natural as puberty. If people can't or won't talk about it, that's their problem. If you can make it normal in your life, not make a big deal out of it, and thus lead by example, you can ease the fears of other women in your life.

We all need to take the drama and the unknown out of menopause. The scariest thing in life is the unknown, so the more we talk about it, the less fearful women will be about it. Chances are high your mother never talked about menopause, which most certainly left you unprepared. Most moms of the previous generation would *never* discuss it! We really need to support each other, since the men in our lives haven't a clue about what's actually going on in our bodies and many of our mothers (or anyone else in their generation) wouldn't talk about it.

Now's our chance to support other women by passing along our knowledge of menopause, just like we pass on knowledge of childbirth.

Next, we'll discuss exercise as a way to not only minimize symptoms but ensure excellent health as you go through the rollicking journey of menopause.

5

EXERCISE

If there's one thing I encourage you to remember, it's this: "Move it or lose it!" Exercise is one of the best ways for you to get through menopause. Exercise will:

- help you achieve and maintain your ideal weight
- strengthen your bones by slowing bone loss after menopause, lowering the risk of osteoporosis and fractures
- reduce the risk of cancer
- reduce the risk of heart disease and type 2 diabetes
- boost your mood (exercise promotes the release of endorphins, one of the body's "happiness hormones")
- prevent cognitive decline
- help treat depression
- help treat anxiety
- reduce stress

- stimulate your lymphatic system, which removes toxins from your body

WHAT TYPES OF EXERCISE ARE IMPORTANT DURING MENOPAUSE?

What's the best workout for menopause? Easy! The best workout is the one that you enjoy. After all, moving your body should be fun!

There's something out there for everyone, whether you join a fitness club, take yoga classes, or work out in your lounge with a YouTube video.

There are several types of exercise that are equally important as you go through menopause: aerobic (cardio), strength, flexibility, and balance. It's easy to slip into a routine in which you're doing the same physical activities every week, but this becomes stagnant after a while. Your body gets used to repetitive activities very quickly. And then you'll find that you're hitting weight loss plateaus, which is especially annoying if you're putting on some menopause weight!

Some sports, like dance, will build your aerobic capacity, strength, flexibility, and balance. However, many sports don't. Cycling, for example, won't build flexibility, so you'll want to cross-train with an activity that does, such as yoga, and do some weight training to build power. You don't need to become the next world-champion powerlifter, but low weights and high reps will work really well. Alternatively, body weight exercises are great, and you don't need a gym membership!

The key is to mix it up and do at least two sports or activities that tick all the boxes.

Aim for a combination of all types of exercise throughout

the week. The best thing you can do for your body is to give it variety. Just like you wouldn't want to eat the same thing at every single meal because you need a variety of nutrients, your body thrives when it's given a variety of activities. Maybe join a new dance class with some friends; if nothing else, you'll have a laugh whilst trying to master the new moves!

Aerobic Exercise

Aerobic (cardio) exercise such as walking, running, cycling, swimming, dance, or aerobics will strengthen your cardiovascular and respiratory systems. Weight-bearing aerobic exercise like running, dance, aerobics, or walking will help strengthen your bones and prevent osteoporosis as you get older. Non-weight-bearing aerobic exercise such as swimming and cycling are great for muscles and the heart, but they should be supplemented by strength training to keep your bones strong.

Flexibility Exercises

Stretching improves flexibility and helps prevent injury. The best time to stretch is when your muscles are already warm, because (and here's a little-known fact) you can actually tear muscles easily by stretching them cold! Stretch after a warm-up and before you do more intense exercise, and then stretch again as part of a post-workout cool-down. Search for a stretching or yoga channel on YouTube and find one you like. Stretches can then simply be done at home in your lounge or bedroom. The convenience of at-home stretches and workouts means you will be more likely to build them into your daily or weekly routine.

Strength Training

Strength training boosts your metabolism by burning calories more efficiently. It builds muscle and helps you shed fat. Strength training will also strengthen your bones and connective tissue, not just your muscles. It can involve body resistance exercises like squats, or it may include hand-held weights or weight machines to challenge your muscles even more. Again, body weight exercises are great for this.

Stability/Balance Exercises

Balance exercises help prevent injury in various sports, and they also help prevent falls. Tai chi, yoga, dance, and racquet sports help develop stability and balance. Exercises such as the plank are also incredibly good at strengthening your abdominal and core muscles.

GETTING MOTIVATED TO START

Ah, this can be the tough part! But below are some tips that are sure to help you:

Start Small

Kami has always been active, but not athletic. Her naturally fast metabolism kept her rail-thin even though she rarely did anything but walk, until...you guessed it. Suddenly, at 51, Kami noticed a belly that hadn't been there before. And her thighs felt softer, even though they hadn't gotten any bigger. Eager to regain her old body, Kami took up running. She decided that two miles was reasonable. For the first two days, everything was great. She was motivated and she was having fun. But then, two days after she started running, she developed delayed onset muscle soreness (DOMS). This is the soreness that hits you a couple of days after you do a new activity, like if you were to go horse-back riding after many years. Kami had no idea that DOMS even existed, let alone what caused it. A few days later she tried again, with the same soreness creeping in after 48 hours. Because she didn't want to feel that beat up ever again, she stopped running. A month later, a friend invited her to a Brazilian dance class. Kami went, loved it, and danced her heart out for several hours. Two days later, she could barely move. This time, she was concerned. Was there something wrong with her? She talked to her doctor, who told her she was okay and that she was just going at it too hard and too fast. Kami reined in her enthusiasm and went back to running, only this time for no more than 15 minutes at a time, which was about a mile at an easy pace, barely faster than a walk. Slowly, she built up her fitness without soreness or injury. Today, at 56, she's in a running club and occasionally participates in fun races. She says, "Don't fall for the endorphin rush when you first start to exercise. Once you feel those endorphins you don't want to stop, but that's going to kick you in the butt, because your body doesn't know what's going on. Go slow to go fast!"

While enthusiasm is wonderful, keep it in check. There are no ways to "get rich quick", so to speak, when it comes to fitness. Start with 15 minutes a day, and check the next section, *Achieving Your Fitness Goals*, on how to set goals that will keep you motivated.

Add "Non-Exercise" Movement

In 2007, a Harvard psychologist conducted a study on mindset and exercise that involved 88 hotel maids. Of that number, 44 of them were told that their job equaled "serious exercise", and the maids were educated on how their jobs made them fit. The other 44 maids weren't told anything. After one month, the maids who'd been told their jobs made them fit had lost weight, developed a healthier body composition (more lean muscle mass), and showed lower blood pressure—even though they hadn't done anything differently with their daily routines or diet! The other 44 maids did not see these benefits.

This shows just how important your mindset is! So then: what types of exercise do you get on a daily basis that isn't considered "exercise"? How about cleaning the house? No? How about speed-cleaning the house as if guests were coming in 15 minutes? Ah...there's some motivation! How about walking the dog? Great! Walk a little faster or further. How about parking as far as possible from the shop instead of cruising around for "rockstar parking" or cycling or walking to the shop?

If you commit to making everyday activities more "active", then you'll set the stage for easily adopting traditional exercise.

Commit to finding ways to make your everyday routine more active for one month. That's how long it took for the Harvard study participants to see measurable results.

Listen To Your Body

You want to push yourself a little, but listen to your body. For example, if you're not feeling up to a workout, identify whether it's your mind talking or your body. As any athlete will tell you, the mind will quit long before the body. If your *mind* is just being lazy, override it! If your *body* is telling you it needs rest, listen to it.

Exercise With Friends

Who better to motivate you than your friends? Chances are you're in the same menopause boat, and exercise is *always* more fun with friends! You can hold each other accountable, motivate each other, support each other when things get hard, and take your mind off your troubles. Exercise is also an opportunity to make new friends!

ACHIEVING YOUR FITNESS GOALS

Don't just say to yourself, "I'm going to exercise more." That's so vague, and it's not very motivational, either! Plus, it sounds so...*boring*. It's not a very enticing goal.

Wherever you are in your fitness journey, success is all about setting the right goals—goals that motivate you. You may have heard of the SMART acronym. There are several similar variations of this, but I like this one:

- **Specific:** Choose an exact weight, clothing size, or fitness goal you want to achieve. Set a goal that makes you feel good and excited just thinking about it.
- **Measurable:** Measurable goals are easier to achieve— a fitness diary or training log can be incredibly motivating as you track your progress and look back on how far you've come.

- **Actionable:** What are the specific steps you can take to achieve this goal? Break down every big goal into steps you can do every day. Small steps really add up fast!
- **Realistic:** You must *believe* that you can achieve this goal. If it's too ambitious, break it into smaller goals that make you feel excited, but not overwhelmed.
- **Timely:** Set a hard deadline for achieving this goal, a reasonable timeframe that's not too far in the future that you'll "start tomorrow" (because no, you won't), and not so soon that it causes stress.

You know the old saying: "It's not about the destination, it's about the journey."

That's true for goals, and it's true for menopause. This is a great time to develop a great relationship with your body or heal your relationship with it. Many of us were never taught to have a good relationship with our bodies. It's such a tragedy that societal pressures made us hate ourselves for having a normal body!

Exercise goals can help you appreciate your body more while coaxing the best out of it.

There are no hard and fast rules to how much aerobic and strength training you should do, because it all depends on your current fitness level, weight, health, and other factors. I recommend you work with a fitness trainer if you're new to exercise. If you're normally active, keep doing it, and remember: this is a new chapter of self-love. Go into this new era of your life with the best body you can, and life will be even more amazing!

Next, we'll talk about how to fuel your body so that you have more energy and fewer symptoms.

6

NUTRITION HACKS TO MINIMIZE MENOPAUSAL SYMPTOMS

Mila went through menopause during a particularly stressful time in her life: she got divorced, which was followed shortly by perimenopause. She discovered early on that she developed an intolerance to caffeine—likely due to chronic stress rather than menopause itself. Instead of being a stimulant, it would actually make her want to sleep more! About three years after menopause, she was able to very slowly reintroduce coffee several times a week.

Many experts recommend cutting back on caffeine during menopause. I know my friend was not a happy girl without her morning brew, so it's important that "you do you." If a cup of coffee in the morning doesn't make hot flashes worse, it'll give you more energy and keep your brain sharper. So it's a trade-off, and individual results will vary.

Keep track of what you eat and drink during menopause. If your hot flashes seem particularly intense after eating spicy foods or drinking coffee, for example, then that's your body asking you to cut back. Some women find that eating a large, heavy meal also makes their symptoms worse.

Fortunately, Mother Nature has provided us with a variety of foods that can help ease our menopause symptoms. And here's the good news: it's not all tofu and yuck!

WHAT TO EAT DURING MENOPAUSE

The best thing you can do for your body as you go through menopause is to take care of your gut health. Keeping your gut microbiota (the gut bacteria) balanced and happy will, in turn, help balance hormones, reduce chronic inflammation, and generally keep your body healthier.

A healthy diet rich in fresh, whole foods and little or no processed foods will do wonders for your gut health. I can't stress enough the importance of getting enough vegetables. This isn't a diet book, but nevertheless, here are my recommendations for foods that will help ease menopausal symptoms.

Foods High in Calcium

Bone loss can accelerate due to lower estrogen production during menopause, especially if you're sedentary. Add these foods to your diet, and consider taking a calcium supplement if your doctor advises:

- Dairy products
- Cultured yogurt or kefir
- Fish
- Leafy greens
- Almonds

- Edamame (young green soybeans)

Micronutrients (Vitamins and Minerals...a.k.a. Vegetables!)

Load up your plate with vegetables. At least half of your food intake should be a rainbow of colorful veggies. For example:

- Leafy greens (lettuce, spinach, chard, kale, mustard greens)
- Cruciferous (broccoli, cabbage, cauliflower, Brussels sprouts)
- Marrow (pumpkin, cucumber, squash, zucchini)
- Root (potato, sweet potato, yam)
- Edible plant stem (celery, asparagus, turnips, kohlrabi)
- Allium (garlic, onion, shallots)
- "Fruity" vegetables (peppers and tomatoes are both technically fruits)

Talk to your doctor about all vitamin and mineral supplements you're considering taking. Some, like magnesium, are said to ease hot flashes. It's important, however, to not fall into the "if some is good, more must be better" trap, and everyone's body is different. In the modern era with so many soils depleted of nutrients, nearly everyone is malnourished to some extent when it comes to micronutrients.

Therefore, a supplement that will benefit one person may throw your own body into chaos, and that's why professional medical advice is crucial. Blood tests can help evaluate your individual nutritional status and will measure the concentrations of essential nutrients and detect nutritional deficiencies.

Vitamin D

It's not fair, but it is what it is: lower estrogen levels weaken your bones. Supplementing with calcium and vitamin D can help slow this process. Good old sunshine is the best way to get vitamin D, but it needs to be balanced with skin health, since the sun will only synthesize vitamin D in the body in the absence of sunscreen! If you're getting 10-15 minutes of sunshine daily without sunscreen, you may reduce your need for vitamin D supplements.

Protein

Protein sources help you maintain bone density and muscle mass—although without exercise, you won't see this effect. Meat, fish, tofu, lentils, nuts, and beans are great sources.

Foods That Increase Estrogen

Some foods are estrogenic, meaning they contain phytoestrogens, which are similar to the estrogen produced naturally in the body. Naturally boosting estrogen, or introducing estrogen-like compounds, can help with hot flashes.

Phytoestrogenic foods include:

- Soy (edamame, tofu, soy milk)
- Seeds (flax, sesame, chia)
- Legumes (lentils, peas, chickpeas [garbanzo])
- Olives and olive oil
- Dark rye bread
- Peanuts

- Fruit (apricots, plums, peaches, strawberries, oranges)
- Vegetables (yams, spinach, broccoli, carrots, kale, celery, alfalfa sprouts)
- Green and black tea
- Culinary herbs (sage, turmeric, thyme)

SUPPLEMENTS TO INCREASE ESTROGEN

You can boost your body's natural estrogen production by supplementing with chasteberry, soy isoflavones, red clover, black cohosh, B-vitamins, vitamin D, DHEA (a naturally occurring hormone that the body converts to estrogen and testosterone), and boron (a trace mineral).

A note on black cohosh: this herb, which is native to North America, is known to help increase estrogen and relieve hot flashes. However, it shouldn't be taken for more than six months at a time, and it may cause stomach upset and diarrhea. Always check in with your doctor before starting any supplements.

Another popular supplement is DHEA (dehydroepiandrosterone, an adrenal hormone), which, among its many functions, makes estrogen in the adrenal glands. Like other hormones, production peaks around 25 and declines steadily with age. Supplementing with DHEA won't boost enough estrogen production to make a difference in vaginal dryness or hot flashes, but it will help you maintain bone density.

Foods That Increase Progesterone

Progesterone is also made up of fat, protein, and cholesterol. Adding healthy fats to your diet can help increase progesterone production.[6]

Other foods that promote progesterone production include beans, cruciferous vegetables, nuts, pumpkin and squash, leafy greens, whole grains, sweet potatoes, and yams.

Nuts

Nuts are rockstars when it comes to raising progesterone. They contain fat, as well as essential hormone-regulating minerals like zinc and magnesium. And they're a great anytime snack instead of sweets!

Dark Chocolate

Here's a free pass: eat dark chocolate. It's for medicinal purposes. The science says so!

Dark chocolate (with at least 70% cacao) is rich in fats and magnesium, which helps regulate progesterone production. This might explain why we naturally crave it before our periods, when progesterone production spikes! So go for it (in moderation, of course).

Yams

Wild yams are believed to increase progesterone. You can also find wild yam extract in the form of a cream that's applied to the skin.

Supplements That Increase Progesterone

Chasteberry, zinc, magnesium, vitamin C, and vitamin B6 have been shown to help increase progesterone production.

The Skinny on Fat

Eating fat will *not* make you fat. If that were the case, the low-fat/no-fat craze of the last few decades would have all of us looking as lean as a 60s supermodel. What contributes to fat gain is excess food, too many carbs, and a sedentary lifestyle. As long as you're moving, as long as the fats you eat are natural (no trans fats!), and as long as you're reducing or eliminating simple carbs (like sweets...sigh) from your diet, eating more fat won't put any extra on your belly or hips.

Aim to reduce carbohydrates (which create a lot of glycogen), as your body will use these glycogen stores as a fuel source rather than targeting your fat stores, making it more difficult to lose the unwanted fat.

Not all carbs are alike, though, so it's good to check out the glycemic index to help you make the best dietary choices. The glycemic index assigns a number to a particular serving of food. The lower the number, the less impact on your blood sugar. Packaged foods should have a glycemic index on the label. There are many sources online that will give you the information you need when you want to reduce your glycemic load for the purposes of weight management and diabetes management. It's worth noting that foods in or close to their natural state often have a lower glycemic index than refined and processed foods.

- 55 or less = Low (good)
- 56-69 = Medium
- 70 or higher = High (bad)

Fat is actually the best fuel you can give your body for sustained energy, or energy that doesn't come with highs and lows like you get with a high-carb (high-glycemic) diet. But not all fats are created alike either, and it's important to choose healthy fats.

So what are "healthy" fats? In the past few decades or so, the emphasis has been on avoiding saturated animal fats, such as bacon or lard, which were labeled "unhealthy." However, recent research suggests that our bodies actually *need* a mix of saturated and unsaturated fats. In other words, if nature made it, it's a healthy fat! With that said, aim for a mix of 90% plant-based and 10% animal-based fats.

And what are trans fats? If you see the words "hydro-genated" or "partially hydrogenated" on a label, put it back on the shelf. These man-made fats are known to contribute to a number of health problems. They're only found in cheap processed foods, and it's a good idea to avoid them anyway.

Be sure to include *natural* fats in your diet (whether from animal or plant sources). Hormones are made up of fat, protein, and cholesterol. This means that women on very low-fat diets actually *reduce* their estrogen production! As well, vitamin D—which you definitely need in higher quantities at this stage of life to prevent brittle bones—is a fat-soluble vitamin. Therefore, if you eat a low-fat/no-fat diet, you'll diminish the amount of vitamin D you're getting.[7]

Healthy fat sources include fatty fish, nuts, olive oil, avocado, flaxseed, soybeans, butter, cheese, and meat.

And remember: cut back on carbs with a high glycemic load as you increase fat intake!

Foods to Limit

Oh, woe is us. Here comes the "sad" part: doing away with the stuff that we love. But wait a minute—let's flip the switch here. Let's realize that these things that we enjoy so much are actually, simply put, terrible for us—especially as we enter and endure The Change. We're doing ourselves a tremendous favor by cutting back or eliminating the following foods to ease menopausal symptoms.

Sugar

Sugar is the #1 contributor to obesity, hormonal imbalances, metabolic syndrome (high blood pressure, high blood sugar, and belly fat), aging skin, and chronic inflammation. If there's one food to stop eating for overall health and easier menopause, it's simple carbohydrates: refined flours, added sugar, and most processed foods, especially low-fat foods (which are loaded with sugar to make them palatable).

Did you know that worldwide sugar consumption has gone through the roof? The World Health Organization recommends no more than 25 grams of sugar per day. And yet the average American eats 126.5 grams per day. Per *day*! Germany and the Netherlands are not far behind us with just over 102 grams per day. Yikes!

And here's the thing: the low-fat/fat-free craze that demonized fats has actually contributed to the obesity epidemic! I've mentioned previously that sugar is added to low-fat foods because without either fat or sugar, they'd taste like cardboard. When you consume excess sugar, your body becomes insulin resistant and inflamed. Inflammation in particular is responsible for all major diseases. It accelerates skin aging and contributes to inflammatory joint disorders.

Here's why this is important: menopause *already* creates inflammation in the body. Estrogen in particular has an anti-inflammatory effect, so when estrogen levels plummet, this hormone isn't around anymore to protect your body from inflammation. A good diet helps significantly and, as I've mentioned, sugar is enemy #1! Simply by eliminating all added sugar from your diet, you'll reduce the inflammation in your body.

Some people like to go cold turkey on all added sugar. This can lead to withdrawal symptoms, since sugar is highly addictive. But in a week or so, you won't crave sugar anymore, and your taste buds will wake up. Even carrots will taste sweet! You can also wean yourself off sugar gradually.

Most added sugar is found in processed food. Read the labels. Say no to sugar, high fructose corn syrup, agave nectar, all artificial sweeteners, and even zero-calorie natural sweeteners. Develop a "spice tooth" instead of a sweet tooth: for example, a sprinkle of cinnamon in your coffee has a wonderfully rich flavor without any sugar.

Trust me: as you give up sugar, your body will respond beautifully!

Caffeine

Excess caffeine (more than four cups of brewed coffee per day) can lead to estrogen dominance. While you might be thinking, "Okay, I kind of *want* more estrogen during menopause", it's the *imbalance* between estrogen and progesterone that can amplify hot flashes and other menopausal symptoms. Estrogen dominance is what you want to avoid, and cutting back on the caffeine is one great way to do this.

Spicy Foods

These can absolutely make hot flashes more intense. Temporarily avoid cayenne pepper, other hot peppers, or pepper products like hot sauce or salsa. To add flavor to your meals, add sage, turmeric, or thyme (which are all estrogenic *and* delicious).

Alcohol

Alcohol can also increase the severity of hot flashes and, especially, night sweats. See if cutting back or eliminating that evening glass of wine with dinner helps.

A Word on Cravings

Indulge your cravings for healthy foods! If you're craving meat, nuts, an avocado, or a simple hummus-and-carrots snack, that's your body asking for specific nutrients. Your body is so masterful at balancing and healing itself! It needs nutritional support to do its balancing act, and you know exactly what it needs when you crave something healthy.

And whatever you do, don't indulge your cravings for sugar (unless you opt for a small bite of dark chocolate or fruit).

INTERMITTENT FASTING: BETTER THAN DIETS!

If you're trying to avoid menopausal weight gain or need to lose a few pounds, I recommend intermittent fasting along with exercise. We all know that diets don't work, not in the long term anyhow. We wish they did, and on the surface the math seems to add up: burn more calories than you eat. However, dieting does something really tricky: it slows your metabolism, which encourages your body to hang on to stubborn fat. That's the last thing you want during menopause, right?

Intermittent fasting, on the other hand, turns up your metabolism, and your body will quickly burn through stored fat.

It involves simply shortening your daily "eating window" by several hours. It's not starvation by any means, since you can eat as much as you'd like during your eating window. Most of us are used to pretty much non-stop eating from morning until bedtime, with rarely more than three to four hours between meals, and often much less because of snacking. This is one of the reasons we gain weight, especially in middle age when we tend to become more sedentary.

Intermittent fasting is a wonderful way to help you maintain a healthy weight through menopause. It also has an incredible number of benefits, including improving gut health, extending lifespan, and balancing hormones.

Researchers observed a group of obese pre- and post-menopausal women for eight weeks. The study participants had a very time-restricted eating schedule, in which they could eat whatever they wanted during a four-hour window, and fasted the remaining 20 hours (this is a very advanced fast and not recommended for beginners, by the way). Another group fasted for 18 hours and had a six-hour eating window. The results for both groups included:

- A modest drop in the hormone DHEA (still within normal ranges at the conclusion of the study), which could help reduce breast cancer risk in pre- and post-menopausal women
- No change in estradiol, estrone, or progesterone
- At the end of the study, the women had lost 3-4% of their baseline body weight
- Both groups saw a decrease in insulin resistance and markers of oxidative stress[8]

Intermittent fasting doesn't involve counting calories or otherwise restricting what you eat, although you'll get much better results if you also stick to eating healthy food. This makes it a lot easier to lose menopausal weight with intermittent fasting than with traditional dieting.

There's a ton of information on intermittent fasting online. Here's the short version, to pique your curiosity:

- If you currently eat three meals plus snacks every day, you're probably eating between 7 a.m. and 9 p.m. (which includes TV snacks after dinner). That means that your eating window is 14 hours, and you're fasting for 10.
- The easiest way to start intermittent fasting is to shorten your eating window to 12 hours by eliminating after-dinner snacks. If breakfast is at 7 a.m., you would finish dinner at 7 p.m. and fast for 12

hours. This is the 12:12 schedule, and already your body is turning to stored fat as fuel.

- Next, you could move up to a 14:10 schedule, in which you fast for 14 hours and eat during a 10-hour window. If you prioritize dinner over breakfast, you could delay breakfast until 9 and finish dinner by 7. If you're very active during the day and breakfast is important to you, you could have your normal 7 a.m. breakfast and finish eating dinner by 5.

- The most popular intermittent fasting schedule is 16:8, in which your eating window shrinks to eight hours a day. Remember, you can eat normally during your eating window, so you never feel deprived. This is when your body is actively turning to stored fat to fuel itself, because it's long since burned through your glycogen stores in the blood and liver. What's interesting though is that you quickly get used to eating normal portions, not larger portions that you believe are necessary to sustain you through a longer fast. This leads to even more weight loss!

If you approach intermittent fasting gradually, it's surprisingly easy to adopt, and there are plenty of online resources to walk you through it.

Anne started intermittent fasting during perimenopause. She says that she went back to her pre-baby weight within a month (after decades of on-and-off dieting), had fewer hot flashes, her skin cleared up, and her joints felt less achy.

I highly recommend you explore intermittent fasting if

you've been struggling with menopause weight gain, or if you just want to boost your health.

Next, let's talk about sex. Contrary to what you may have heard (or even felt!), sex is a part of life that doesn't have to pack up and leave with your childbearing years!

7

MENOPAUSE AND A SMOKIN' HOT SEX LIFE

J ust because you can't make babies anymore doesn't mean you can't keep the fire burning! Whether you're in a relationship or single, you may be worried about how menopause affects your sex life. Like everything, sex may be different now, but that doesn't mean it's a has-been!

At 54, Meghan fell in love. She was very nearly finished with menopause when she met Aaron at a neighborhood party. She wasn't looking for a relationship, but the two clicked. She hadn't taken HRT and was worried that vaginal dryness would be an issue. To Meghan's surprise, there were no problems in the bedroom. She'd educated herself on what to do in the case of vaginal dryness or painful sex. Her solution was simply more foreplay—and having lots of lube on hand!

Menopause could very well be the beginning of a new chapter in the bedroom. You may need to devote extra attention to your body, but you do that for *you* anyway so that you can feel confident and attractive.

Not all women experience a lower sex drive as they go through menopause. Some actually say their sex drive improves!

Heidi laughs, "My poor husband! He doesn't know where this sex-crazed cougar came from. He keeps asking where I was 20 years ago, to which I reply, 'I was chasing little kids around while trying not to get pregnant every time you looked at me!' He says he wishes he still had a young man's sex drive so that he can keep up!"

A libido boost in menopause may be linked to less anxiety about becoming pregnant, as well as fewer child-rearing responsibilities, which free up time for women and their partner. We've also touched on the fact that testosterone levels decrease very, very gradually throughout our adulthood, whereas estrogen drops like a bomb. This means that when your testosterone levels are higher than your estrogen levels, you might feel a bit more amorous! Another factor may be that older men know how to delay their satisfaction. If they go longer, your interest may be stronger, too. And finally, at this age, you know your body, you know what you like, you know what your partner likes, you know what turns you on. It's not uncommon for menopausal women to have more orgasms than younger women (who may f&@% like rabbits, but rarely take the time to make sex the incredible feast for the senses that it can be as we mature).

For most women, libido often declines during menopause and sexual activity plummets (according to one study, fewer than half of post-menopausal women are sexually active).

Judging by what's going on in our bodies during menopause, nature didn't intend for menopausal women to be sexually active, at least not for reproductive reasons. But we're not a species of animal that only has sex when the female is in heat. We do it for fun!

There's simply *no rule* that says you can't, or you shouldn't, enjoy this wonderful aspect of life. There are things you can do physically, emotionally, and even medically to keep your love life spicy through menopause and well beyond. While many women become dissatisfied and even disinterested in sex during menopause, *you don't have to be a statistic.*

Again, everyone's different. Menopause may lower or increase your sex drive. If you're "on fire", then go get some! And if you're struggling, here's what can help.

TIPS FOR A BETTER SEX LIFE IN MENOPAUSE

Your mind is your most powerful erogenous zone, psychologists say. With that said, we can't deny the role that our changing bodies play in our desire for sex. Below are some ways to keep your love life spicy through menopause and beyond.

HRT

Hormone replacement therapy can boost libido, vaginal tone, and lubrication. However, it's not a quick fix. When low estrogen levels make the walls of your vagina thin and less elastic, sex is probably going to hurt. Topical estrogen—given as a cream, suppository, or ring—can help increase vaginal wall thickness and elasticity. It can also help with increasing lubrication. Most sources say the effects become noticeable within three to six months after starting HRT.

Go Easy on the Antidepressants

This one is tricky. You don't want to feel miserable, so you take antidepressants. But those antidepressants often destroy your libido. Serotonin reuptake inhibitors like Prozac treat depression, but they're notorious for squashing sexual desire. Other antidepressants like Wellbutrin have less of a libido-destroying effect. Talk to your doctor if you need to treat depression *and* you want a satisfying sex life.

Other ways to manage depression are exercise, being in nature, a strong community, and a sense of purpose.

Manage Stress

Relationship issues, family pressures, job stress, financial worries, and menopause-related stress can put sex at the bottom of the priority list. Make stress management a top priority and you may see a boost to your libido.

Try Libido-Boosting Supplements

According to Harvard Health, supplements like ginkgo biloba, ginseng, fenugreek, horny goat weed, Tribulus, yohimbine, and maca are herbs that boost female libido. Zinc is also said to help. In addition, one of the world's most popular aphrodisiacs is the spice saffron. While these effects may be due to increased blood flow or the placebo effect, does it matter if it works? But remember to go easy on supplements: just because something is labeled "natural" doesn't mean it's safe, especially if you're taking any medications. Do your research and talk to a holistic health care practitioner, herbalist, or traditional Chinese medicine doctor to learn more about herbs and other supplements that can boost your libido.

Play Up the Foreplay

If you're not as easily aroused as you used to be, you're not alone. But this doesn't mean that those embers can't be coaxed into a roaring flame! Arousal depends on many factors, including blood flow to your vagina and clitoris. Spending more time on foreplay helps prepare your body for sex—and it's a time to really connect with your partner!

Add Pheromones

Pheromones are chemicals produced by the body that trigger a sexual response in others. As we age, we produce less. Studies are few and mixed, but if you like, you can add pheromones to lotions, body oils, perfumes, and other products. Whether it's the pheromones that make you more attractive to a partner (or a potential partner) or whether you just *feel* more attractive because of them (and therefore put out the "come hither" vibe), who cares? If it works, it works!

Raise a Glass to Love

A glass of wine can be a powerful aphrodisiac. Just don't overdo it!

In a slightly different approach, make sure you're well-hydrated throughout the day so that every cell in your body, especially the ones in your genitals, are plumped up and not shriveled like little half-empty water balloons. Yes, it's a gross visual, but it's intended to drive home the fact that many of us are chronically dehydrated, which actually interferes with cellular function and health. This may help with vaginal tone and elasticity, too—and you'll also notice that your skin looks more youthful.

Play Up the Fantasy

Many women report that indulging in a fantasy during sex helps them enjoy sex more, and that it helps them to reach an orgasm. Reading erotica together or watching a steamy movie can help you and your partner get in the mood.

Use a Warming Oil

Massage oils that create a warning sensation in the genital area can increase arousal and satisfaction. Any oil, including coconut or olive oil, can heighten those fiery sensations. They're messy but worth it!

Have Fun with Toys

Clitoral stimulation devices and other adult toys can be useful when vaginal intercourse is too painful. In fact, just becoming aroused through the use of these devices can stimulate natural lubrication.

Be Liberal with the Lube

Vaginal dryness is a common menopausal symptom, and it's actually the one easiest to manage; it's effects can be eased with silicone- or water-based lubricants, or good old coconut oil or olive oil. If you're still having periods and your partner is using condoms, *do not* use petroleum jelly like Vaseline, which will degrade condoms and render them useless.

Experiment

Some positions may be less painful and more pleasurable to you than others, and we're all different! One woman I talked to can only climax in the cowgirl position (she on top, facing him), but this has been her situation since well before menopause! If you suddenly find that a favorite position isn't doing it for you like it used to, mix things up and try something new.

Also, remember that sex doesn't even have to be about vaginal penetration! Erotic massages, oral sex, and manual stimulation are all amazing ways to enjoy the big O!

Some couples report that changes to sexual routines is a huge boost to their sex life, so shake things up!

Work with Your Partner

If vaginal dryness, poor body image, and loss of libido are making things awkward in the bedroom, remember something I mentioned much earlier in the book: men go through something similar to menopause, something called andropause. He may experience some of the same symptoms you do, although not as dramatically. Men's testosterone levels drop gradually—

not in one giant explosion like ours, so their bodies can more easily adapt to the decrease. But we all know the biggest detriment of low-T that a lot of men deal with as they age: erectile dysfunction.

Keep in mind that a good sexual relationship takes two, and it all starts with communication. Talk to your partner if your libido has dropped. Menopause may add a layer of difficulty to sexual intimacy that was already on the rocks, so the sooner it's dealt with, the better. Also, don't fake it! Communicate with one another, and you'll reap the rewards in the sheets.

More than likely, he's feeling insecure about his sexuality, too! I've found that talking it out over a glass of wine, or in the car so that you can avoid awkward eye contact, is a great way to clear the air. You can approach it in a non-threatening, non-confrontational way. Something like, "I'm feeling terrible about myself, and I'd love to talk to you about it. I don't need you to fix it, I just need you to hear me out."

You may need to compromise if one of you wants more frequent sex than the other. Even couples who've had great sex throughout their relationship may find that things are changing, so you're not alone. Try recreating the atmosphere or the situation that led to the best sex of your life, and don't be afraid to try new things together!

You shouldn't have to suffer in silence or have an unsatisfying sex life. Constant communication is vital for healthy relationships. If it's just too awkward to talk about, seeing a couple's therapist could help. Seeing your doctor about vaginal dryness and other symptoms can help, too. You may be prescribed HRT if your symptoms make sex painful. And some women, if they don't want to take HRT, use a natural lubricant like coconut oil. Hey—if it works, do it!

If your partner is feeling rejected because of your low libido, it needs to be discussed. A partner who feels rejected may not want to initiate sex, which can, in turn, make the other partner feel rejected, too! Don't let these feelings fester.

For many women, spontaneity gets buried under responsibilities, and so even if they're feeling amorous, they push it aside in favor of "adulting." I highly recommend making a date with your partner and putting it on your calendar, because intimacy *should* be a priority. If this is too structured for you and you think, "I can't just turn it on whenever it's convenient", then make the date a special getaway. A whole weekend away, just the two of you doing things you love, can be the spark that lights the fire!

More than anything, go out and live life together, because boredom is a libido destroyer. Travel, do things you both love, laugh, have date nights, and be silly with one another. If you have kids and they're grown and gone, that means that it's just the two of you and it's the perfect time to rekindle the flames.

Always remember that both of you are in the same boat when it comes to aging. It may manifest in different ways (erectile dysfunction, vaginal dryness, low libido, etc.), but it does exist for both men and women to some degree. The best remedy is to adjust your expectations and approach life with humor!

And if you're one of the lucky women whose libido goes through the roof during menopause, you may run into the problem of a man who can't keep up with your increased desire. There are worse things in the world! But, again, communication is key.

Before you get out there on the dating scene, take care of the menopausal symptoms that are most bothersome, whether it's vaginal dryness, low libido, or hot flashes. Remember that HRT is a popular remedy for symptoms that can interfere with a healthy sex life.

Having the right partner helps (a lot) to prime your body for sex. But there's no shame in getting help so that you can still enjoy this aspect of your life without hesitation!

HRT won't rekindle a waning sex drive, but the right partner can. New relationships mean a tsunami of hormones and chemicals like oxytocin and dopamine, which do a lot for your libido. Having the support of a little extra estrogen in your body will also prime it for sex!

Remember that just because you can't get pregnant once you're menopausal (though you can if you're perimenopausal!), you can still get sexually transmitted diseases. The same personal protection rules against STDs apply now as when you were in your 20s!

So let's talk about finding a good partner. In her childbearing years, a lot of a woman's drive to find a partner was driven by the biological urge to procreate. Now that childbirth is off the table and you're entering this new chapter of self-love, be sure to choose a partner who is truly worthy of you. Many women at this age find that they're looking beyond physical characteristics. They're looking for a true partner, and, often, the sexual attraction grows as you get to know each other, even if the initial sexual feelings aren't as intense as when you were both younger.

You could also play the cougar card and date younger men!

Plenty of younger men are attracted to older women. And hey—if society thinks it's okay for men to date younger women, it's absolutely okay for you to do the same if you like. You can teach them a thing or two, and they'll make you feel smokin' hot. Dating younger men is most often a short-term situation; younger men will often eventually want to settle down with a woman closer to their age, but maybe not. If the connection is there, it's there!

IF YOU'RE NOT HAVING SEX (WITH A PARTNER)

Some of us find ourselves in the situation of not having a sexual partner. Whether it's a stale sexless marriage, not finding "Mr. or Ms. Right" (or "Mr. or Ms. Right Now"), or a personal choice, it's still important to enjoy sexual satisfaction as we go through menopause.

Regular sexual activity by self-stimulation can help keep your vagina elastic and lubricated. It also helps keep your mental and emotional "juices" flowing. There's absolutely no reason not to feel good sexually as you age, even if you're taking matters into your own hands!

HELP YOUR BODY FEEL SEXY

How you feel about yourself is the #1 thing that will make you attractive to potential partners. Confidence shows, and so does self-love. How you feel about your body shows up in the way you dress and present yourself to the world.

So love yourself! Do what it takes to build confidence about your body: get to a weight and shape you like with exercise and a healthy diet, accept yourself, and always remember that beauty comes from the inside!

Some psychologists say that your libido is all in your mind anyway. Try relaxation exercises (it's hard to get turned on when you're stressed) and visualization (indulge some daydreams of those steamy fantasies) to put yourself in the mood.

Kegel exercises will keep your hoo-ha as firm as it was before childbirth. Empty your bladder first, and then squeeze as hard as you can (as if you had to pee really bad in the middle of giving a keynote speech) for 5-10 seconds. Relax, and do another set of reps. Repeat daily—even in a meeting if you want; no one will know (and they might be doing it, too)! Pro tip: Kegels make meetings go faster!

I've mentioned that a wardrobe makeover can do wonders for your psyche. Again, it's not about dressing sexy, but about dressing elegantly so that you *feel* like a million dollars. If you feel good about how you look, it's much easier to get turned on!

8

LIFESTYLE HACKS TO HELP YOU ENJOY MENOPAUSE

The previous chapters have been focused on the physical aspects of menopause. I hope that by now, you're feeling well prepared for what's to come and how to deal with it. The emotional aspects of menopause are a bit tricky.

Elizabeth is 63. She had a very difficult menopause emotionally, as The Change coincided with a divorce and a business failure. For Elizabeth, menopause was the final straw, with powerful symptoms. She says, "John left me with crushing debt. My shop closed. And just when I thought I couldn't take any more, here comes menopause. Like, what the hell? My brain was Swiss cheese. I couldn't sleep. I had night sweats. I put on 20 pounds, and I'm certain most of that weight was water from the tears I cried. Worst thing, I became someone I never thought I'd become. A bitch! I was lashing out at everyone. Not a day went by when I didn't shout at someone or cry—and usually both. I started losing friends because I was so awful to be around. I didn't even want to be around myself. Finally, I realized that I needed help." Elizabeth found relief with antidepressants, but because of pre-existing conditions, she wasn't able to take HRT. "Once my depression and anxiety were under control, I realized that the hot flashes and brain fog weren't as bad as I made them out to be when I was at rock bottom. At that point, I just threw my hands up and said to myself, 'This is nothing compared to the tornado that John left in his wake.' Putting it into perspective helped. If you have a lot going on, menopause is the least of it. If you have nothing else going on, you are a magical unicorn!"

Connie is 52. Her children are "grown and flown." She's excited about this new chapter of her life now that she has time for her own interests. Outside of her thriving career as a financial planner, she's looking forward to learning pottery and she's signed up for a creative writing course. She also joins her husband in volunteer projects several times a month. Connie's remedy for menopausal symptoms is simple: "Keep busy doing what you love to do. The busier you are, the less time you have to dwell on your body." Connie is a woman with a lot of bubbly energy. You'll rarely see her sitting still, even in the evenings when most people are relaxing in front of the TV. She doesn't believe that she's unique in being so energetic. She says, "There's just so much life to live! I can't wait to get up in the morning. At work, I get to serve some amazing clients, then I go to the gym, and I spend my evenings enriching myself. This gives me energy. Having a purpose always gives you energy."

For many women, menopause *finally* presents an opportunity for self-care. I'm not talking about indulging in a bubble bath every evening if that's not your thing—but if it's your idea of the perfect evening, do it! Let's dive into some of the ways you can show yourself some love as you enter menopause.

How do you manage the stresses of life? If you're feeling gloomy or irritable, check in with yourself. Is it menopause, or is it "life"? Even though menopause doesn't cause depression, it seems to coincide with growing depression in some women, especially those who've had depressive episodes in the past. As I've mentioned, many of us feel overwhelmed because there's just so much going on in our lives. And, being women, we naturally tend to put others first.

Knowing effective ways to relieve stress can be the difference between struggling and suffering through menopause, and thriving through it. Below are some favorites I've gathered over the years:

Mindfulness Meditation

This practice is associated with fewer (and milder) symptoms of menopause, especially in women who are under a great deal of stress.

Mindfulness meditation involves focusing your attention on this very moment: the thoughts, the sensations, the experience —and observing the present moment without judgment. There are many ways to get your mind out of the past (with its nostalgia and its regrets) and out of the future (with its uncertainty, hopes, and fears). Right now is the only reality; after all, the past and future only exist in our imaginations. That's why the saying "be here now" is so important. We miss out on so many delightful moments when our thoughts are stuck trying to relive the past or racing ahead to the future!

To slip into a meditative state, simply hold your focus on

something until your mind and body relax. You could stare at a candle flame, listen to music with a repetitive beat (and no lyrics to distract you), or sit by a rushing creek or waterfall.

Rachael, 59, used to be a meditation instructor. These are her favorites:

> Close your eyes and slightly, without straining, cross them and imagine you're looking out through your third eye (the point just above and between your eyebrows). Hold your attention there and breathe deeply. Rachael says that when she first tried this, her mental chatter stopped completely!
>
> Do the box breathing (mentioned earlier): inhale to the count of four, then hold for four, then exhale for four, and finally hold for another four. That's one cycle. Do as many as you like. You can do this to the beat of a song, the rhythm of footsteps, the ticking of a clock, and other rhythmic sounds.[10]

Engage Your Senses

Pay more attention to the little things. It's such a cliché expression, but "stop and smell the roses" really is good advice. When you eat your next meal, engage *all* your senses, not just your eyes and mouth. Slowing down and savoring the little moments in life brings immense happiness and calm. Life is nothing but a collection of little moments, and it's a shame to let any of them pass unnoticed.

Breath Meditation

Pay attention to the experience of breathing—how your breath moves in through your nose and into your lungs, the rise and fall of your chest and belly, the small pauses between inhales and exhales, and how the inhales can feel cooling and the exhales warming. Even a minute of breath-focus whenever you're stressed or overwhelmed can help so much!

Body Scan

Wherever you are, whatever position you're in, check in with your body. Scan your body from your toes on up to the tip of your head. Notice any sensations, including pain, and be aware of any emotions or thoughts that come into your awareness.

Walking Meditation

Walking meditations are great for those of us who have trouble sitting still. We always tend to start fretting about our to-do lists, but walking meditation helps. To practice it, go wherever you like to walk, wherever you feel peaceful. Begin walking slowly. Immerse yourself in the experience of walking, just like you immerse yourself in the experience of breathing. The experience of walking includes feeling the ground under your feet, noticing how the air feels on your skin, the sounds of the environment around you, the quality of the light, any aches or sensations in your body, the cadence of your breathing, and even the feel of the clothing you're wearing.

Notice how your body is so good at orchestrating many

different muscles to enable you to walk. It's such a complicated process, yet we do it so effortlessly and often, without conscious thought! It's truly amazing how stress melts away when you check in with your body about something you do unconsciously most of the time.

Curiosity Meditation

When you have a hot flash or notice any other symptom of menopause—or any strong emotion—really lean into the experience. Recognize the prickly heat, the flushing of your face, the sweat beading up on your forehead, the weird crawling sensations, the chills, the elevated heart rate, and so on. This helps you to experience a hot flash or strong emotion without becoming upset about it because you're too busy being curious at how the heck your body went from normal to nuclear in a matter of seconds! Ride out the physical sensation until it fades naturally, which it will, in a matter of seconds or minutes.

If You Don't Enjoy Traditional Meditation, Try This

If meditation is not your cup of tea, or if you get stressed out just thinking about sitting and doing nothing, it's okay.

There are other ways to reap the benefits of meditation. You don't need a lot of time, you don't need any special training, you don't have to pretzel yourself up into a Lotus position, and you don't have to light incense.

Have you ever stared, absolutely mesmerized, into a fire? The dancing of a candle flame, a crackling fire in a fireplace, or the under-the-stars experience of a campfire? Yes, it's like "Caveman TV"—you just can't stop watching! If you've had that experience of totally immersing yourself in the flames and can't take your eyes off them—then you have meditated!

Light a scented candle or fill the room with candles and lose yourself in the dancing flames. Wine and bubble baths are optional, but highly recommended.

Here are two meditations that can help you if you find it impossible to sit still.

Be In Nature

Getting some fresh air and sunshine are great for your body and your attitude. Make it a point to spend at least 15 minutes every day outdoors, and you can accomplish two things at the same time: a little exercise and a little attitude adjustment.

Remember way back in Chapter 2 I mentioned that the color green is a natural antidepressant? It can even be used to treat migraines. No wonder we feel so good when we're outside! Wherever you live, make it a point to get close to something natural and green every day. Yes, potted plants count, but try to get outside, like a park or a neighborhood where people take pride in their gardens and landscapes.

Luisa is a busy executive with a lot on her plate. She uses her lunch breaks to walk in a local park while listening to podcasts or audiobooks. The walk leaves her energized for the afternoon, and she also enriches her mind at the same time.

If you're not a type A personality who's always on the go, try to take nature at a slower pace. Again, be here now. Take notice of the miraculous ways that nature operates. Everything has cycles and rhythms—just like your body.

Listen to Music

Philosophers say that music is the language of the soul. You may need to dance around the house to loud rock music one day and relax with some chamber music the next.

Your emotions influence your outlook, and a single song can completely change your emotions. It's a powerful tool!

Charlotte has three playlists on her phone: Work Out Jams, Chillax, and Happy Dance. What about you? Does your life have a soundtrack? Music can help you dance through menopause— whether it's a graceful waltz, a sexy samba, or, like Charlotte says, "Whatever boy band you're still listening to in secret, because we all have one whether we admit it or not."

Take Up a Hobby

What activity do you enjoy that absorbs you to the point where you don't hear the doorbell ring? Do more of that. Now is the time to hone your skills and master that hobby, and even turn it into a career if you want!

Elizabeth discovered glass painting at 53. She'd never considered herself an artist, but she was fascinated with the process. When painting on glass, you work backwards: the details in the front are applied first, and then you gradually move backward. So the leopard's spots are painted first, and then the leopard! It's not an easy skill to master. Elizabeth dove into glass painting headfirst as a way to occupy herself as her kids left home. She credits the focus and "reverse engineering" with keeping her mind sharp during menopause.

Prioritize YOU

Many women give and give and give to others, and they tend to put themselves last. I can relate! Menopause can be a time where you shift your focus onto yourself. I know, I know...you still have a million responsibilities no matter what your life situation is! But menopause can be a wake-up call: "Take care of *me*" for a change!

What prioritizing yourself means for you is so very individual. One thing that's almost universal for women is to learn to finally say no more often. Do it with kindness and without lengthy explanations, but do it. Especially if you haven't felt comfortable saying no in the past, it's important to prioritize yourself and your needs and wants. People may not be used to hearing no from you, but they'll get over it.

Build a Community

Having a community of supportive people is critical at any point in your life, and certainly during menopause. Of course, girlfriends who are going through menopause at the same time can be your best source of comfort, because they truly get what you're experiencing.

For many women, menopause coincides with an empty nest and a shift in social circles—one that corresponds with rekindled or new interests, and social activities that don't revolve around the kids. In a way, these are the friends we choose. We don't know them because they're our partner's workmates. We don't know them because they're our kids' classmates' parents. We know them because they share our interests and values.

9

FINDING PURPOSE: THE ART OF SELF REINVENTION

In this chapter, I'd like to introduce the concept of menopause as a superpower. When you think about how brief your fertile years were—say, from 13 to 40—that means that the rest of your life is actually longer than those child-bearing years, whether you had kids or not. It's a bit shocking to put that into perspective, because we place so much emphasis on being young and sexy without realizing that most of our lives, we're not (at least, not in the way that society wants us to be).

This makes us kind of special, despite what narrow-minded men like Sigmund Freud said: "It is a well-known fact...that after women have lost their genital function, their character often undergoes a peculiar alteration" and they become "quarrelsome, vexatious, and overbearing."

So basically, according to Freud, we become men when we stop menstruating? Ha! the joke's on you, Sigmund!

Those insufferably sexist doctors, the Wilsons and Freuds, made some truly demeaning and pompous statements about how useless women become as their childbearing years come to an end. Unfortunately, this has tainted the way we are seen by society, and I say it's time to change that!

We can learn from the animal kingdom. In most species, females rarely live much past their ability to give birth, but whales are different. Orca females who are no longer raising young become matriarchs, guiding their pod to the best hunting grounds. They become leaders.

In traditional societies, too, the matriarch is important. Older women have the life experience to not only care for grandchildren and pass down family traditions, practical skills, and knowledge, they can also provide for their families: in the Hadza tribe of Tanzania (a modern hunter-gatherer society), postmenopausal women are the best foragers, often bringing home far more than they need to sustain themselves and their family.

It could be that calling menopause a "syndrome" or a "disorder" is intended solely to take away a woman's power in the years when she becomes the most powerful. But conspiracy theories aside, now is your time to roar!

One of the most inspiring stories I've heard is about Helena, a menopausal woman who refused to lie down and die. She's a woman who decided to do a complete career change. At 60. She actually went back to her roots, which were in architecture and design—a wild change from her long career as a copywriter for a marketing firm! She'd always loved design, and she realized that she was at her absolute happiest when she was designing and renovating every home she'd lived in as an adult. After the third complete home overhaul (the third house, not the same one), she had the lightbulb moment that this is what she should be doing with her life. This is what made her consistently happy. This challenged Helena and gave her purpose. In high school, a misguided guidance counselor insisted that Helena's math grades weren't good enough to go into architecture. Crushed, she pulled away from her dream. After college, after having worked as an administrative assistant at an architectural firm, she realized that, in fact, basic math skills were more than adequate, and so she went back to school for architectural design. Then life got in the way again. She got pregnant, and this time deliberately put her career aspirations on hold because she wanted to be a full-time mother. As she went through menopause, she decided that it was now or probably never! This time, she focused on interior design, and back to school she went! She's now a successful interior designer, and I've never seen her so alive!

The Change can often be seen as a springboard for personal transformation, or even complete reinvention of who we are. As women, we're expected to give, and then give some more. Many of us lose small parts of ourselves as we enter into a marriage and have kids, or as our careers take center stage. Now is the perfect time to reclaim *who you are*. One of the benefits of menopause is that we often *finally* become comfortable in our own skin. We can look at the anxiety that plagues 20- or 30-year-old women, because those anxieties don't apply to us anymore. We're more mature. We've been around the block a few times and we've lived a lot. You see, even though menopause is often described as a loss of our looks and sexuality, *my goodness* we were immature back then! Today we're much more balanced, emotionally stable, and wiser. We're better able to prioritize our lives according to our higher aspirations, not just our reproductive drive.

I encourage you to get in touch with what makes your heart sing. Is it something you loved as a child but gave up because others pulled you away from it? Isn't it time to get back to that original passion? After all, you're the adult now. You get to decide what you do!

What makes you want to jump out of bed in the morning? Do more of that! Even if you don't make a career out of it, just having a sense of purpose can help you make this chapter of your life the most rewarding.

Ask yourself this: how would your life look if you spent just 15 minutes a day devoted exclusively to something that makes your heart sing?

For most of her life, June called London her home. She raised a family and ran several small shops there. After her kids left for university, June felt she needed a change. Her desire for something different coincided with menopause. Her symptoms were often so bad that she'd have to hide out in the back of the shop and let her assistant deal with customers. So June decided to move to the countryside and do what she'd always wanted: write children's stories. Her reasoning was that she would be less stressed, and she wouldn't have to deal with embarrassing hot flashes in front of customers. June's menopause journey was a difficult and lengthy one. She refused HRT, which may have helped, and while her approach of moving to the countryside won't work for all of us, it was right for her. In the process of learning to manage her symptoms, June discovered meditation. And, like life often does, this led to a new passion and ultimately a career—this time as a meditation teacher. She's even opened her beautiful home as a summer meditation retreat. She says, "Don't sit home with nothing to do, because then all you can think about is how miserable you are. Get out! Do something with yourself! Feel good!"

When you think about it, humans are creative beings. It's who we are! We're always making things! This doesn't mean we're all *artists*. Finding solutions to a problem is a creative outlet. Doing something to inspire others is creative, too. What are you good at? What do you find so easy and take for granted that other people find difficult? Do more of that!

You may find that you have more time for yourself in this in-between stage of caring for kids and caring for aging parents. If that's your situation, embrace it. It's a time of freedom (possibly the only time in your adult life). Make this chapter all about your own passions and talents. This is an opportunity to put your passions and talents to use in making *your* world a better place.

Volunteering is one way that many women find a sense of purpose. You may think that you don't have the time to devote to serving your community, but there are infinite ways to help. Find an organization whose work you admire, and ask them what they need. You might be surprised!

And on this same topic, remember that learning to say no more often will give you more freedom to be you. You'll have more time, less stress, and less frustration when you prioritize yourself!

WELCOME TO "CHAPTER WONDERFUL"

Menopause is a time of massive change. For some, it can be a tough passage, while others have an easier go of it. Most of all, it is a time of choice. It should be a time of allowing yourself to be you, freely and unabashedly.

Most of all, maintain a positive and empowered attitude toward menopause. It's not the end—it's a transition to a new beginning! I'm not in any way implying that you should not mourn the passing of your reproductive life; by all means, do what feels right! But don't wallow in the past. How you approach menopause will hugely affect your experience. Today is an opportunity to show the world that you still have gas in the tank and that you still have a lot of love to give and a lot of life to live.

I hope this book has prepared you for the closing of one chapter and the opening of another. I hope you've learned a lot. I hope I've eased your concerns, helped you know what to expect, and showed you how to prepare for menopause.

I hope you laughed a lot too, and that you feel a sistership with the women in this book. These are all real stories (though the names have been changed), and it's my wish that you feel empowered by them!

I'd like to leave you with a smile on your face with a few more funny stories from women who've learned to laugh in the face of The Change and all the hilarity it can bring.

Robyn: "I drove to the spot where I usually take my dogs for a walk. I had my boots on and had the leashes and poo bags and everything we needed, and when I opened the car to let the dogs out..."Where are the dogs? There are no dogs in the car!" I'd forgotten to take my own dogs on their dog walk!"

Elisha: "I once texted my husband to tell him he'd left his phone at home."

Katerina: "Last week, I went out to work with one navy and one black shoe one. I didn't realize until a colleague told me."

Dana: "Recently I was ranting to myself, 'Who the hell took the margarine? Someone must have put it in the bin!' I turned the kitchen over looking for it. I'd put it in a pan, in the pan cupboard. Of course! Why would it be anywhere else…'"

Larisa: "I was sitting on the sofa and the neighbors talking outside. I couldn't hear what they were saying, so pointed my TV remote at them to try to turn the volume up. Fortunately, they didn't see me."

Erin: "Once when I was icy, I turned the heater on in my car to defrost the windows. I left it running and then spent another ten minutes trying to find my car keys that I'd ten minutes earlier left in the ignition to keep my car running."

Melissa: "Yesterday, I emptied a pouch of cat food into the bin rather than the cat's bowl. He didn't like that too much."

I'd keep adding more, but can't remember them at the moment…

To me, the funniest thing about menopause has been the laughter. There are so many women out there who know *exactly* what you're going through. It may seem sometimes that we've been transported into a different body that doesn't fit quite right, and then we have to learn all about its quirks. But, in the process, we can learn to love our new bodies—and we can also learn to laugh about menopause together!

If you've found this book helpful, I'd appreciate a review on

Amazon! Don't forget to order the tracker/journal to help you keep a log of all your symptoms.

I wish you all the best in this sometimes-frustrating, some-times-funny, but always-interesting new chapter of your life! Remember—it's not the end. You've only just begun!

PHYSICAL SYMPTOMS

Physical Symptoms of Menopause:

- Hot flashes
- Night sweats
- Irregular periods
- Vaginal dryness
- Decreased libido
- Fatigue
- Insomnia
- Weight gain
- Hair thinning or loss
- Dry skin
- Breast tenderness
- Joint and muscle aches
- Urinary incontinence
- Urinary frequency
- Urinary tract infection

- Dry eyes
- Allergies or sensitivities
- Vertigo
- Soreness after sex
- Cravings
- Bloating
- Water retention
- Itchy skin
- Blurred vision
- Floaters in eyes
- Shaking (jitters)
- Dizziness
- Burning tongue
- Metallic taste in the mouth
- Tinnitus (ringing in the ears)
- Dry mouth
- Headaches and migraines
- Sensitivity to light and sound
- Changes in the sense of smell
- Changes in body odor
- Brain fog
- Forgetfulness
- Loss of concentration
- Restless legs
- Bleeding gums
- Bad breath

EMOTIONAL SYMPTOMS

Emotional Symptoms of Menopause:

- Mood swings
- Irritability
- Anxiety
- Depression
- Fatigue
- Difficulty concentrating
- Memory lapses
- Brain fog
- Feelings of sadness
- Crying spells
- Restlessness
- Feelings of loneliness
- Decreased self-esteem
- Lack of motivation

- Increased sensitivity
- Easily overwhelmed
- Loss of interest in previously enjoyed activities
- Anger or rage
- Frustration
- Decreased patience
- Emotional instability
- Changes in sexual desire or satisfaction
- Feelings of loss or grief
- Loss of a sense of purpose
- Lack of confidence
- Nervousness or jitters
- Feeling emotionally detached
- Feelings of being invisible or irrelevant
- Fearfulness or phobias
- Panic attacks
- Increased sensitivity to criticism
- Feeling on edge or easily startled
- Worry or rumination
- Feeling overwhelmed by responsibilities
- Difficulty making decisions
- Feelings of guilt or shame
- Changes in appetite
- Emotional cravings for certain foods
- Feelings of emptiness
- Increased need for reassurance
- Social withdrawal or isolation
- Difficulty adjusting to life changes
- Vivid dreams or nightmares
- Feelings of uncertainty about the future

- A sense of being out of control
- Difficulty coping with stress
- Increased self-consciousness

HOLISTIC REMEDIES FOR MENOPAUSE

Suggested Holistic and natural alternatives to help relieve Peri-menopause and menopause symptoms. However, don't overwhelm your body as it transitions through this new balance of hormones.

Do your own research along with keeping lines of communication open with your Doctor prior to making any changes.

Suggested lifestyle adaptations :

1. Healthy Diet including lots of fruit and vegetables
2. Exercise regularly
3. Keep well hydrated
4. Getting Proper Sleep (6-8 hrs per night)
5. Stress-Reducing/Mind-Body Practices
6. Reduce refined sugar and processed food
7. Stop smoking
8. Yoga

Be aware of potential interactions of any herbal supplements before you apply an holistic approach to relieve your symptoms. Always **seek medical advice** first.

Supplements and Herbal Treatments. The following can help with :

1. Vitamin D – vaginal dryness and boost mood
2. Soy – hot flashes, vaginal dryness, night sweats
3. Wild Yam – mimics estrogen
4. Milk Thistle – hormonal balance, mood swings and anxiety
5. Sage – hot flashes, mood swings, brain fog
6. Maca root – hot flashes, uninterrupted sleep
7. Sea Buckthorn – vaginal dryness, itching and burning
8. Coconut oil – vaginal dryness
9. Vitamin E – Skin dryness and irritations
10. Agnus castus- PMS symptoms, hot flashes, night sweats
11. Red clover – lower fat in blood
12. Evening primrose oil – hot flashes
13. Magnesium – maintenance of strong bones
14. Ashwagandha – balancing mood and night sweats

BIBLIOGRAPHY

[1] Whiteley J, DiBonaventura Md, Wagner JS, Alvir J, Shah S. The impact of menopausal symptoms on quality of life, productivity, and economic outcomes. J Womens Health (Larchmt). 2013 Nov;22(11):983-90. doi: 10.1089/jwh.2012.3719. Epub 2013 Oct 1. PMID: 24083674; PMCID: PMC3820128. https://www.ncbi.nlm.nih.gov/pmc/articles/PMC3820128/

[2] David Lowe, 2011, Mechanisms Behind Estrogen's Beneficial Effect on Muscle Strength in Females, doi: 10.1097/JES.0b013e3181d496bc

[3] Song He, 2021, The Gut Microbiome and Sex Hormone-Related Diseases doi: 10.3389/fmicb.2021.711137

[4] Angelo Cagnacci, 2019, The Controversial History of Hormone Replacement Therapy, doi: 10.3390/medicina55090602

[5] "The Experts Do Agree About Hormone Therapy," 2023, The North American Menopause Society

[6] Sunni Mumford et al, 2016, Dietary fat intake and reproductive hormone concentrations and ovulation in regularly menstruating women, doi:10.3945/ajcn.115.119321

[7] D. Bagga, 1995, Effects of a very low fat, high fiber diet on serum hormones and menstrual function. Implications for breast cancer prevention, DOI: 10.1002/1097-0142(19951215)76:12<2491::aid-cncr2820761213>3.0.co;2-r

[8] "How intermittent fasting affects female hormones", 2022, Science Daily https://www.sciencedaily.com/releases/2022/10/221025150257.htm

[9] "Reproductive Horomones", n.d., Endocrine Society. https://www.endocrine.org/patient-engagement/endocrine-library/hormones-and-endocrine-function/reproductive-hormones

[10] Elordi, Jon. 2020, jonelordi.com. https://www.jonelordi.com/james-nestor-breathing-techniques/

ABOUT THE AUTHOR

Grace Rose was born and raised in Manchester, UK. Family, friends and fun are at the heart of everything she does. This prompted her to write:

"Menopause? Hit Play, Not Pause!"
"A Wise Woman's Guide to "The Change"

Grace has a degree in Health and Sports, and has always enjoyed the benefits of a fully functioning body and mind. She worked as a PE teacher in a secondary school for many years. Her passion was teaching Physiology and understanding how the body works. Therefore when her body started to 'malfunction', Grace immediately researched the possible reasons this may be happening.

Research showed she had now stepped into the next stage of her life; the menopause years, Yikes! Being the mother of two young adult daughters, Grace decided not to listen to the horror stories and instead allow her fun and humorous take on life to approach this 'Change' with laughter and understanding.

Grace is now a full-time property investor which allows her more free time to sit in her farmyard summerhouse overlooking the fields where her husbands sheep and cattle graze, and write away to her hearts content.

Printed in Great Britain
by Amazon

31776565R00084